Children
of Prenatal
Substance Abuse

School-Age Children Series

Series Editor
Nickola Wolf Nelson, Ph.D.

Children of Prenatal Substance Abuse
Shirley N. Sparks, M.S.

What We Call Smart: Literacy and Intelligence
Lynda Miller, Ph.D.

Whole Language Intervention for School-Age Children
Janet Norris, Ph.D., and Paul Hoffman, Ph.D.

Children of Prenatal Substance Abuse

Shirley N. Sparks, M.S.
Western Michigan University

SINGULAR PUBLISHING GROUP, INC.
SAN DIEGO, CALIFORNIA

Singular Publishing Group, Inc.
4284 41st Street
San Diego, California 92105-1197

© **1993 by Singular Publishing Group, Inc.**

Typeset in 10/12 Palatino by CFW Graphics
Printed in the United States of America by BookCrafters

Library of Congress Cataloging-in-Publication Data

Sparks, Shirley N. (Shirley Nichols), 1933–
        Children of prenatal substance abuse / Shirley N. Sparks.
            p.   cm. — (School-age children series)
        Includes bibliographical references and index.
        ISBN 1-56593-071-1
        1. Children of prenatal substance abuse — Rehabilitation.   2. Drug
abuse in pregnancy — Prevention.   3. Alcoholism in pregnancy —
Prevention.   I. Title.   II. Series.
        RJ520.P74S7   1992
        618.92'86 — dc20   92-28621
                                                                                       CIP

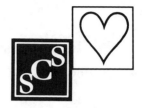

Contents

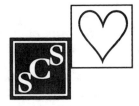

Foreword

When children enter school they enter a whole new world. The acquisition of the spoken and unspoken rules for communicating in school and in life beyond school is a major focus of the school-age years. However, not all children experience "normal" development, including normal communicative development, in the same ways. The books in this series are designed to help speech-language pathologists and other special education professionals, teachers, and parents to collaborate with each other and with children as they attempt to acquire the skills needed for success in school and in life.

Each book in the series is designed to educate readers about a particular area of concern and to engage readers in problem solving to reduce the need for concern. Although grounded in theory, the books are applied in focus. Several themes unify the series. First, collaboration is consistently viewed as a desired mode of problem solving. Second, children are seen as individuals whose needs are shaped by multiple contexts that change over time and across situations and cultures. A third unifying theme is change — both change among children with problems and change in the important contexts of their lives. The final unifying theme is relevance. All volumes are aimed at helping professionals become more relevant in meeting the real-life needs of children.

Shirley Sparks' book, as the inaugural volume in the series, establishes the tradition. The problems of children affected by their mothers' substance abuse are a primary concern to all of society as the turn of the century approaches. As Sparks makes clear, the problems such children experience are not theirs alone; they justify a united, collaborative approach from the rest of us, including teams of professionals with diverse expertise.

Sparks deftly introduces the problems of children affected by substance abuse in a way that permits readers to balance outrage over preventable problems with concern about individual children and the real people who are their parents. Professionals are guided to confront their own ingrained attitudes on one level; on another, they are guided to understand the rationale for gathering substance abuse histories and to acquire realistic strategies for doing so. Interventions are considered for children who were exposed in utero to alcohol and to cocaine and related drugs. Communicative expectations are emphasized, but children are viewed as whole systems functioning within and affected by larger educational and family systems. Research results (where they are available) are presented and interpreted to guide professional practice, and the federal requirements of P.L. 99-457 and the Individuals with Disabilities Education Act (IDEA) are presented as mechanisms for encouraging collaborative, family-based problem solving modes. Sparks provides a review of available literature and assists readers in understanding the problems of data collection from her own experience.

It is this experience that makes Sparks' contribution particularly special. As a colleague, I have not only watched Sparks teach fellow professionals to understand the problems of children affected by substance abuse, I have watched the sensitivity with which she addresses those needs herself. Whether it is helping young mothers tune in to their babies or young professionals to know what questions to ask, Sparks conveys a sense of caring about the process and the people involved. It is that sense of caring that is perhaps the most important quality conveyed in this work. I am pleased to introduce it.

Nickola Wolf Nelson, Ph.D.
Series Editor

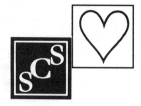

Preface

Dr. Marshall Becker, much revered professor at the University of Michigan's School of Public Health, taught me the difference between a pioneer and an adapter. A pioneer, he said, is the first to try something new — the first to have an idea and the one other people look to for advice and information on a subject. Adapters, on the other hand, are people who take the ideas and information from the pioneers and help to diffuse them throughout a population.

This book is the result of my attempts to be an adapter whose purpose is diffusing the ideas of some pioneers in the field of substance abuse to the population of school personnel and service providers. Some pioneers have contributed through painstaking research; others have contributed through trial-and-error hands-on intervention. Dr. Ann Streissguth, University of Washington, has long been a pioneer in fetal alcohol syndrome and fetal alcohol effect research. Not only has she written extensively, but she has translated her results into meaningful recommendations for interventions. Her colleague, Dr. Donna Burgess, has pioneered curricular interventions for children with FAS and FAE, and her work has been a valuable contribution to this book. Dr. Ira Chasnoff, National Perinatal Association Research and Education Association in Chicago, is likewise a pioneer in maternal cocaine and polydrug exposure. He, like Dr. Streissguth, not only has conducted the pioneering research in his field, but also is skilled in sharing that information with those of us who work with children who are exposed prenatally to drugs and with their families. I have also relied extensively on the research work of Dr. Dan Griffith, who, with Dr. Chasnoff, has followed the progress of a cohort of children exposed to various drugs. It is their work that has given us the best information we have on long-term effects of maternal cocaine and polydrug exposure.

That there are so few pioneers only points out the scarcity of our knowledge. The work of the pioneers must be replicated with other cohorts of children and parents. The difficulty of that research is daunting, as is pointed out in Chapter 8, but it must be done. On the other hand, we cannot wait for research to give us "truth" because the children who must be served are in our schools today.

In this book, each affected child is seen as part of a family: in a dyad with a caregiver and in a larger family system. Other pioneers have brought insights into working with families that are necessary to working with a child and his environment, but the caregiver and family affected by substance abuse impose different problems for us as intervenors. The chapters on the nature of addiction and the unique problems of working with families affected by substance abuse are meant to help school personnel understand those special problems. Perhaps more important than understanding substance use and abuse on an intellectual level, the reader is asked to understand his or her own feelings about substance use and abuse and how we view those who use substances while pregnant. I did not say those who "choose" to use substances, because that is usually not the case. Women do not choose to use drugs after they become pregnant; rather they become pregnant while they are using drugs. A major contributor to understanding the relationship of a woman and the drug(s) she uses is Dr. William Schafer, former president of the Michigan Association for Infant Mental Health. I have relied extensively on his powerful writing in the chapter on working with the substance abusing family.

I have asked a great deal of my readers: to understand addiction and drugs; look critically at the research; base your interventions on the research; evaluate your programs; work to get the children eligible for Part H funding; collaborate for best service delivery. Additionally I have asked you to help prevent these disorders which are 100% preventable. It is not enough to assess and treat the children; we must do what we can through prevention to keep this tragedy from happening.

As a speech-language pathologist, my focus has been on the cognitive and communicative functions of children prenatally exposed to drugs. I have generally approached behaviors as communications. However, the book is not meant only for speech-language pathologists. It is hard to imagine any function in which communication is not important for all of us. From the interactions of infant and caregiver to employer and employee, communication is at the root of our social being. By the same token, all of us and all the children with whom we deal are in families. Substance abuse is so common that it is a rare family without an affected member, which in turn affects all the personal relationships within that family. For those reasons, this book is intended for school personnel and service providers — regular education teachers, special education teachers, counselors, speech-language pathologists, early interventionists, social workers, health providers, and administrators. To quote Donna Burgess and Ann Streissguth (1992), "If we focus on team-building, both within and among our disciplines, we can make progress toward creating effective programs."

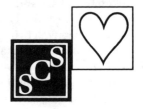

Acknowledgments

A number of people have been directly helpful to me as I prepared the manuscript and to whom I owe thanks: Dr. Nickola Wolf Nelson, the editor of this series, for asking for this contribution and for her valuable suggestions; Dr. Michael J. Clark, my colleague at Western Michigan University, for his careful review of the manuscript; Sandra Lopacki, Northwestern Memorial Hospital, Chicago, for sharing her experiences; Dr. Izuru Takeshita, University of Michigan School of Public Health, for teaching me about program evaluation; and the parents, who, by sharing these stories of their own children, have contributed to our understanding of how prenatal exposure to substances affects children.

I also wish to express my heartfelt thanks to my wonderful children and friends whose constant and steadfast support and encouragement sustained me through my work on this book.

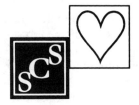

Prologue

I have watched Jeffrey grow up because he is a member of my extended family. His parents, both professional people, adopted him at the age of 5 weeks. He was the second of their two adopted children; a few years later they had a natural child.

It was obvious to his mother by the first week that something was wrong with this baby; he cried nearly all the time and continued to cry for the first 3 years. He did not eat a lot, but there were no feeding problems. He slept very little. When he learned to walk, he walked on his toes a good deal. One of his first "words" was "B.M.," much to everyone's embarrassment and his delight. He repeated it over and over and giggled. Masturbation was a problem very early. His facial features as a child were classically fetal alcohol syndrome (FAS): hypertelorism, flat philtrum, small head, and long face, but at that time — he was born in 1964 — FAS was practically unknown. He was extremely hard to care for by parents who had easy babies both before and after him. As an adult, he calls himself a "sex addict" (heterosexual). He remains small and of slight build.

Jeff's school life was a succession of disasters. At the end of third grade, his parents were told by school officials that they did not want him in the public school. He was too disruptive. He constantly clapped his hands and seemed out of the teacher's control. Punishment had no effect on him then, or ever. Private school of some kind was the only option his parents had. If they had not been able to afford it, one wonders what would have happened. His parents found a military school that would accept such a young child, and he went there from grades four to six. He got into trouble there: The bigger boys sent him out to buy cigarettes for them, and he was caught. He did not realize the consequences of his actions and was easy prey for exploitation. He went back to his home town for junior high and high school but by 10th grade he was in constant trouble at home and at school. As his mother said, "He was so close to normal that we couldn't give up. If he had been retarded or even easy to love, we would have accepted it — and dealt with it." Numerous physicians, psychologists, and educators were consulted. There were no answers, but one psychologist said he would never be able to hold a job or live on his own.

When he was in 10th grade he became abusive to his sister and brother, and his parents looked for somewhere else for him to live. Relatives on a farm in a nearby state volunteered to have him live there and finish school. It did not work out, and he was off to another military school. He graduated there with the designation "most improved cadet." He thought he would like to try college and enrolled for a summer while living in the home of an instructor there. He received one C and two Ds and college seemed to be out. That fall he headed to a city where there were lots of jobs in the entertainment industry. He could always find work as a busboy, waiter, bill collector, errand boy — all of which bored him. He lived in a succession of places where he skipped out without paying. He spent most of his income on obtaining sex. He began lying and stealing, even from his family, at an early age. He seemed to have no conscience. He never had a drug problem and has always been very conscious of good health. He seemed to crave love and affection, but was viewed by all who knew him as unlovable.

What about the signs of FAS that we as service providers and educators look for? Some of his school history follows a typical FAS pattern; but, as with every case, there are exceptions. He did not have ear infections. His speech and language seemed to develop on schedule, but he had some trouble with sequencing. His reading comprehension and spelling were not a problem, but he had such difficulty taking written tests that his ninth grade exams were give orally. He could do arithmetic in his head and liked algebra. His attention span was very short, and he could not stay on task long enough to complete his homework.

Jeff is now 27 years old. He has both a full- and a part-time job. The maximum time he has held a job is 2 years. He longs for marriage and a family, but his attempts at relationships have not ended well. He knows, and has known for a long time, that he is not like other people. He has made several appointments for counseling but has broken them. His relationships with his family members are troubled. Jeff seems to be hanging on in life, but his parents fear that disaster may strike again — that there will be another phone call that he is in trouble or that he did not think through the consequences of his actions yet another time.

Would Jeff's life have been different if he had been identified as an at-risk child because of FAS? If he were starting school today, a number of interventions might have made life better for him and his family.

- Fetal alcohol syndrome would be identified as a cause, giving both Jeff and his family a reason for his problems.
- The Individual Family Service Plan process would have identified his family's need for information and provided counseling about what to expect from him.
- Early intervention would have helped him and his family with their interactions. Perhaps his early challenging behavior could have been modified. Perhaps, too, he and his parents could have learned to interact in ways that would have rewarded all concerned.
- He would not have been asked to leave public school. An unanswered question is whether a classroom for learning disabled or for attention deficit disordered children would have been preferable over military school, where he seemed to have the best experiences of his life. A program for FAS children would be ideal, but even today Jeff might have been placed in a classroom for emotionally disturbed children instead.
- Perhaps his extreme sexual behavior could have been modified with counseling. A school program that helped him with job skills and social skills would have been in order.

We have not come as far as we would like in our interventions for children like Jeff who have been exposed to alcohol prenatally, but when we look back on this child and his parents, trying to cope with a baffling problem for which they could not get help, it seems that we have come a long way since Jeff was a child. In the following pages, we will discuss the current state of research and knowledge about addiction and the drugs of addiction, how service providers deal with emotions surrounding substance abuse, how prenatal substance abuse affects children, guidelines for designing and evaluating intervention programs, guidelines for preventing prenatal substance abuse, and some recovery treatment issues for women.

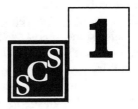

Understanding
Substance Abuse

Dr. Ira Chasnoff, a pioneer in prenatal substance abuse research, opens his conferences for professionals in this manner:

> Suppose that you and a friend are taking a walk downtown on a beautiful spring Saturday, and you are doing some window shopping. You see an alcoholic coming toward you. You know it's an alcoholic because the alcoholic is stumbling all over the sidewalk. You and your friend look at each other. You are both a little uncomfortable so you move closer toward the window side of the walk. You stop and pretend to look into a window to avoid interaction. You smell alcohol and avoid any eye contact as the person goes by. Finally, the alcoholic passes by and you and your friend breathe a sigh of relief. (Chasnoff, 1992)

As you imagined yourself in the above situation, what image did you have of the alcoholic? Chances are that you saw, in your mind's eye, a skid-row bum — the stereotypical alcoholic on the street. Chances are slim that you envisioned a female alcoholic or pregnant woman, even though you have chosen to read a book about the effects on children of prenatal substance use by their mothers. It is certainly not unusual, then, that other professionals, including physicians, perceive the typical substance abuser as someone other than a pregnant woman. The reasons for this perception are deep-seated in our feelings about women, pregnancy, alcohol and drugs, and addiction.

Treatment has developed in a dichotomous fashion among professionals; some of us treat the mothers and some of us treat their children, and it is possible that we may not cross paths. Those of us who treat children could possibly fall into the trap of thinking of the mother as no more than a reproductive vessel. Perhaps the emotion that most describes our feelings about a mother who uses substances while pregnant is anger. She certainly has not fulfilled expectations of the mother's nurturing role in any contemporary culture. How could she do such a thing, particularly when so much public education is available about the dangers of drugs and alcohol during pregnancy?

Eventually, all the infants and children affected by substance exposure are in the schools. This book is written for the school-based service provider who has substance-exposed children in his or her caseload, which includes nearly all of us. It is also intended as a resource for other members of the early intervention team and for those school personnel designated as "child finders" — those to whom referrals are made and who then implement assessment and intervention services. Child finding is not confined to only these individuals, however. A speech-language pathologist, classroom teacher, social worker, nurse, psychologist, or home visitor may be the finder. The child is part of a family system, and it is a mistake to think that providers or child finders can take a child out of a family system to do evaluations and interventions and then return him or her to it when finished (Trout & Foley, 1989). Good professional practice requires that we assess and treat a child in the context of his or her family, and if that family is affected by drug use, we must be knowledgeable about drug and alcohol use and be willing to take the steps necessary to serve affected children.

In this chapter, some questions about the dynamics of addiction will be addressed. We may need to work with a mother, who is either still using substances or who is in recovery, in order to treat her child. In either case, we must deal with her behavior and our expectations about her behavior. School personnel may know little about the process that produces a child affected by prenatal substance abuse. Our own anger and hostility that a child is affected who need not be, no matter how well it may be submerged, will not serve that purpose well. Some common questions are: What makes a woman abuse substances when she is pregnant? What are women like who use drugs? What are the signs of substance abuse? When a drug-using woman stops, why does she relapse?

The drugs discussed in this chapter are alcohol and cocaine, the two that are of most interest at this time. Other drugs (opiates, PCP, benzodiazapines [Valium], nicotine) also have suspected or substantiated fetal effects, but a full discussion of all addicting drugs is beyond the scope of this book. Children exposed prenatally to alcohol or cocaine will be referred to as *substance-exposed children.* A substance-exposed child may or may not be *affected* by that exposure. Disorders that result from alcohol exposure are *alcohol-related disorders.* The term will include both fetal alcohol syndrome (FAS) or fetal alcohol effect (FAE), terms that differentiate severity of disorder, as explained in Chapter 5. There are no terms to differentiate severity of disorder in cocaine exposure. A withdrawal syndrome has not been identified; therefore, at this time it is inaccurate to describe a cocaine-exposed newborn as crack-addicted (Zuckerman, 1991). "Crack babies" and "addicted babies," terms coined by the media, connote that the child is marked for life. Such terms are inaccurate, and they are resented by both professionals and family members.

◼ DRUG ABUSE

The definition of drug abuse depends on societal *attitudes* as to what constitutes abuse. It is not synonymous with addiction or dependence. Jaffe (1990, p. 522) gives drug abuse a social definition: "the use of any drug in a manner that deviates from the approved medical or social patterns in a given culture." Thus, one drug may be perceived as being abused in some situations, but not others (e.g., alcohol is not acceptable at a school function but is acceptable in a private home); and other drugs may be perceived as abused if used at all (cocaine). In other words, we have a sliding scale about use or excessive use and how that use relates to inappropriate behavior. That sliding scale incorporates the user's gender. Our perception of motherhood is that we do not want to believe that a pregnant woman would use any kind of drugs that would be harmful to her baby.

Other definitions of drug abuse take into account the *pattern* of use. The American Psychiatric Association (1987) identifies three criteria that must be met to diagnose substance abuse. This definition stresses medically inappropriate behavior and attaches a time limit to it.

- ◼ a pattern of pathological use
- ◼ impairment in social or occupational functioning caused by the pattern of pathological use
- ◼ duration of at least one month

Other terms are used to refer to patterns of drug use: *experimental drug use* (one or a few times because of curiosity, peer pressure, scientific interest); *recreational (casual) use* (moderate use for pleasure); *circumstantial use* (for specific purposes occasionally, for fatigue, for instance).

◼️◻️ ADDICTION

Addiction is a relatively vague term that "is used to connote a severe degree of drug dependence that is an extreme on a continuum of involvement with drug use" (Jaffe, 1990, p. 523).

There is a difference between drug abuse and addiction, and there are women who are drug abusers, but who are not addicted. For women who are drug abusers, prevention efforts targeted at giving them information on the effects of drug use on the fetus can be effective. It might be difficult to change those habits, but it does not pose the degree of difficulty that it has on the addicted woman. The addicted woman is most difficult to understand and most difficult to change. Certainly people take drugs (and alcohol is included as a drug) because those drugs are reinforcing in some ways. To understand addictive properties of drugs, and in turn how to break the cycle of addiction, it is helpful to understand why they are reinforcing. One of the strongest predictors of addiction is the degree of reinforcement derived from the first experience with the drug.

Dependence

When a person is addicted to a drug, he or she is said to be dependent on that drug. Alcohol and cocaine produce different types of dependence. Alcohol produces *physical dependence.* Physical withdrawal symptoms, which are the opposite of the drug effect, occur when the drug is discontinued. Alcohol is a sedative hypnotic (see Chapter 5 for alcohol's mechanism of action). One of the effects of sedative hypnotics is to depress seizures, and seizures may occur on withdrawal. A mild withdrawal symptom is a hangover, but severe physical symptoms of withdrawal can be serious or even life threatening.

Physical dependence is not necessary for addiction, however. Cocaine does not produce physical dependence, although a few physical signs may be found on withdrawal, yet it is highly addictive. Cocaine is a psychomotor stimulant (see Chapter 3 for cocaine's mechanism of action). Psychomotor stimulants are excitatory and induce a feeling of well-being, as well as depressing the urge to sleep. On withdrawal, addicted persons are depressed and have difficulty sleeping, but the symptoms are not life threatening. The dependence is *psychological:* nonphysical symptoms upon withdrawal are characterized as intense craving for the drug, which the user thinks is absolutely necessary for well-being.

Tolerance

The development of *tolerance* often leads to people taking higher and higher doses of a drug, which increases the likelihood that dependence will develop. Tolerance occurs when more of the drug is necessary to maintain the drug's effect. Put another way, it is necessary to increase the dose of a drug to maintain the same effect when the drug is given repeatedly (McKim, 1991). An individual may also build tolerance to another drug in the same class by becoming tolerant to one drug, which is referred to as *cross-tolerance.* Thus, people who are tolerant to alcohol become cross-tolerant to barbiturates and other sedative hypnotics, and those tolerant to cocaine are cross-tolerant to amphetamines and other psychomotor stimulants.

Reinforcement Effects of Drugs

Most service providers are familiar with theories of reinforcement. Two hypotheses are used to explain the reinforcement effects of drugs (Robinson, 1991, personal communication): negative and positive reinforcement.

Negative Reinforcement

Drugs are taken to alleviate the negative (physical or psychological) symptoms that people experience when they withdraw from the drug. The main problem with the negative reinforcement hypothesis is that it does not explain why addiction develops in the first place — just why it is maintained. Furthermore, it does not explain why relapse is so prevalent after withdrawal symptoms are over. Addicted persons may resume their drug habits years after becoming drug free. Most drug treatment professionals expect relapse to occur in treatment. Relapse does not mean that sobriety will not be achieved in the long run.

Even after enrollment for prenatal care, addicted women are not likely to maintain sobriety. MacGregor et al. (1987) noted that only one third of their patients were able to maintain a drug-free state after enrollment for prenatal care. Achieving and maintaining sobriety carries a complex set of stresses for a pregnant woman: she must leave her previous life and perhaps her family, she may have few resources, and, if she can find a treatment program that accepts pregnant women, it may not have transportation or child care.

Positive Reinforcement

Drugs are taken for the state they induce (euphoria) instead of the state they alleviate. It feels good, and the memory of that is sufficiently powerful to lead to drug-seeking behavior. One reason that positive reinforcing effects continue to control behavior is that they are experienced immediately after behavior, whereas the punishing and painful effects are often delayed. A well-understood principle of operant conditioning, which we use in therapy, is that if a consequence is delayed, its ability to control behavior is diminished. Thus, if a drink of alcohol causes pleasure within minutes and a hangover causes discomfort a number of hours later, the pleasure rather than the hangover is more likely to determine whether the person will drink again. When punishing consequences occur infrequently and after a considerable delay, no matter how severe they might be, they are less likely to exert as much control over behavior as immediate gratification (McKim, 1991). However, the positive reinforcement model does not explain how people can continue to take drugs in the face of extremely punishing circumstances. Addicted individuals will continue taking drugs when the consequences could hardly be more negative: the loss of one's family, job, and even life. Among those punishments are the effects on the fetus.

Competition from Other Reinforcers

The above explanation is overly simplistic. Many other factors contribute to the addiction equation. One of these is competition from other reinforcers. Under normal circumstances there are numerous reinforcers, both positive and negative, in the environment that influence behavior: positive reinforcers such as food, social recognition, money, water, or sex; and negative reinforcers such as pain and social rejection. In an environment where the influence of positive reinforcers is minimized because they are difficult to achieve or unavailable, the impact of introducing a new reinforcer — such as a drug — might be considerable, and it could easily come to dominate most behavior, especially if the drug is readily available and inexpensive. Once this dominance is established, the effect may be difficult to reverse. Thus, environmental nonreinforcers such as boredom, poverty, and lack of social support may contribute to the strength of drug abuse (McKim, 1991).

In some cases, the use of a drug can diminish opportunities to obtain other reinforcers and therefore contribute, either directly or indirectly, to even more drug use. Use of alcohol, for example, can disrupt relationships with one's spouse or interfere with work and thereby diminish reinforcement normally available from the family or the workplace. This diminished availability of reinforcement can lead to more drinking. Factors such as these can also contribute to relapse in former drug users. It has been shown, for example, that recovering alcoholics are more likely to return to using alcohol when there are disruptions in work and family life (Vuchinich & Tucker, 1988).

So far we have looked, albeit superficially, at the part reinforcement can play in addiction, but questions remain: Why does the pattern of drug-seeking and drug-taking in some individuals become a progressively more all-important and compulsive activity, at the expense of all other activities, including mothering? How can a drug be so important that it can support day-long hustling and determine a whole subculture? Why is it such a struggle for a mother to maintain sobriety when she has made a commitment to sobriety and keeping her children may depend on it? Two other concepts are important in answering these questions: the concept of addiction as a disease and the concept of environmental conditioning.

Disease Concept

Only in the 20th century have drug use and abuse been studied systematically. Before that, people who had trouble with drugs were considered to be deficient in character, moral fiber, will power, or self-control. Consequently, addiction to drugs was a problem for clerics rather than scientists to understand. When society's definition of drug abuse changed from being a moral to a medical problem, it became the object of scientific investigation.

According to Jellinik (1960), "A disease is defined as follows: In general, any deviation from a state of health; an illness or sickness; more specifically, a definite marked process having a characteristic train of symptoms. It may affect the whole body or any of its parts, and its etiology, pathology, and prognosis may be unknown" (p. 11). He cites scientific writings dating from 1937 about alcoholism as both a psychological and a physical disease. Alcoholism is defined as: "A chronic, progressive and potentially fatal disease characterized by tolerance and physical dependency or pathologic organ changes, or both. All are the direct or indirect consequences of the alcohol ingested" (National Institute on Alcohol Abuse and Alcoholism, 1981).

A more contemporary disease model (George & Marlatt, 1983) has four basic assumptions:

- Alcoholism is a unitary, identifiable phenomenon.
- Alcoholics and prealcoholics differ from nonalcoholics in important constitutional factors. This difference exists prior to alcohol use and manifests itself in the form of alcoholic drinking behavior when the person is exposed to alcohol.
- Because of "loss of control," abstinence is the only goal of treatment intervention.
- The alcoholic is a helpless victim of internal physiological mechanisms beyond his or her control.

The disease model fits well with the observation that some people become addicted and some do not in the way that a disease may afflict some and not others. It also means that an addicted person requires treatment and not punishment. However, the woman who drinks to excess or uses drugs is still stigmatized; she is seen as morally deficient and an object of scorn, rather than the victim of a disease. This double standard has had a profound effect on the ability of a woman to seek help for her disease, or to be helped by those close to her. It should be noted that even though the alcoholic is said to be powerless over alcohol, she or he is thought to have it within her or his power to do something about it. Nearly all treatment programs focus on the addict being responsible for taking the necessary action to get over the addiction.

Are some people more susceptible to the disease of addiction because of their genetic makeup? Considerable interest has been focused on the genetics of alcoholism and drug abuse. Whereas few scientists can dispute that heredity can create a susceptibility to alcoholism (Horgan, 1992), relatively little is known about genetic influences in other types of drug abuse. This disparity is directly related to the amount of research that has been done in the two areas recently (Pickens & Svikis, 1991). Hill and Smith (1991) have suggested that early onset female alcoholism, although rare in the population, may well be a more severe form and is likely to have a genetic component.

Environmental Conditioning

A situation of high risk for relapse is when a person returns to the same environment in which drug-taking took place. Recent psychological literature strongly supports the theory that taking drugs in a particular environment causes the drug taker to be conditioned to that environment. In other words, the environment in which one takes drugs becomes a conditioned stimulus, and when the user is placed in that environment again, the environment acts as a "primer" for taking the drugs, and previous withdrawal symptoms may even appear. According to Stewart, de Wit, and Eidelboom (1984):

> The fact that re-exposure to the environment, previously associated with drug-taking, often leads to relapse in experienced, but drug-free, individuals, even after prolonged periods of abstinence, suggests that drug-related stimuli acquire the status of conditioned incentive stimuli and gain the ability to prime behavior just as unconditioned or primary incentives do. (p. 254)

Addicts who have been drug free for long periods of time are drawn back to drugs when placed in the environment where drug-taking took place. As the following example illustrates, there can be little doubt that these conditioned withdrawal symptoms play an important part in relapse to drug use in postdependent addicts (O'Brien, 1976).

> The patient was a 28-year-old man with a ten-year history of narcotic addiction. He was married and the father of two children. He reported that, while he was addicted, he was arrested and incarcerated for six months. He reported experiencing severe withdrawal during the first four or five days in custody, but later, began to feel well. He gained weight, felt like a new man, and decided that he was finished with drugs. He thought about his children and looked forward to returning to his former job. On the way home after his release from prison, he began thinking of the drugs and feeling nauseated. As the subway approached his stop, he began sweating, tearing from the eyes, and gagging. This was an area where he

had frequently experienced narcotic withdrawal symptoms while trying to acquire drugs. As he got off the subway he vomited onto the tracks. He soon bought drugs and was relieved. The following day he again experienced craving and withdrawal symptoms in his neighborhood, and he again relieved the symptoms by injecting heroin. The cycle repeated itself over the next few days and soon he became readdicted. (p. 533)

■□ WOMEN AND ADDICTION

Women do not *start* to abuse drugs when they become pregnant; rather they become pregnant while they are using drugs. They may have every intention of quitting their drug use when they become pregnant, but they may not suspect pregnancy in its early stages. Missed menses can be interpreted by the addicted woman as a result of drug use and not conception. As a result, addicted pregnant women tend to seek help during their third trimester rather than during the first or second trimesters (Daghestani, 1988).

Polydrug Use

Any discussion of drug use, whether for men or women, must also consider the combined effects of drugs. Polydrug use is more common than the exclusive use of one drug. The majority of cocaine users also use marijuana, alcohol, and cigarettes (Chasnoff, 1988). Street drugs are often "cut" with other substances. Another drug can also be used to lessen the effects of the primary drug and offset the "crash" after the extreme high of cocaine, or to prolong the high. When I collected data for the research project described in Chapter 9, I took drug histories from more than 20 women. The form listed the drugs that I thought were used, including cocaine, crack, pot, heroin, and alcohol. The first few women whom I asked about crack answered negatively to the question about pot. Then when I asked about *how* they used crack, the chosen method was in a "primo" — a marijuana cigarette with a small rock of crack in it. The women who used primos did indeed use marijuana, but they did not think of themselves as marijuana users. Women addicted to alcohol often use more socially acceptable substances, such as tranquilizers, sedatives, and amphetamines, before they start to drink, and they may continue to use them while they are drinking.

Profiles of Impairment in Women

Addiction in women can result in impairment of physical health, mental health, and social functioning, all of which have an impact on pregnancy and parenting (Bennett, 1992).

Physical Health

The chaotic life style of the drug culture is not conducive to compliance with prenatal care visits and regimens or to obtaining sufficient nutrition during pregnancy. General medical histories of drug users may include anemia, multiple infection, hypertension, general lack of medical care, menstrual dysfunction, decreased fertility, hepatitis, adult-onset diabetes, urinary tract infections, or chronic undernourishment (Daghestani, 1988). Obstetric histories may include spontaneous abortion, premature labor, precipitous delivery, abruptio placentae, low birth weight, and fetal distress. Pregnancies may be characterized by inappropriate weight gain, an inactive or hypertensive fetus, fetal tachycardia, and unusually strong contractions early in labor (Schafer, 1989). The incidence of tuberculosis, once thought conquered by public health measures, has risen sharply in the last few years, primarily in the drug culture. Prostitution, to obtain money for cocaine, puts women at high risk for sexually transmitted diseases: gonorrhea, trichomoniasis, chlamydia, syphillis, and HIV infection. They are also at increased risk for HIV and AIDS if they share needles or have a sex partner who does.

Alcoholic women are at risk for alcohol-related illness (e.g., liver disease, gastritis, pancreatitis, heart disease). Streissguth, Clarren, and Jones (1985) found that mothers of infants with FAS are often hospitalized during the infant's first years of life, and a disproportionate number of them die of alcohol-related causes while the FAS children are still young. Thirty-eight percent of the mothers they studied, whose whereabouts were known, were dead before the children were 6 years old. The prediction of high mortality rates for alcoholic women is borne out by studies of other populations cited by Blume (1986) in which their mortality rate was four times greater than expected, and their life expectancy was decreased by an average of 15 years. Frequent causes of death include suicide, accidents, violence, cirrhosis of the liver, cardiovascular ailments, and malignancies.

Mental Health

Only a small percentage of addicted women would qualify for treatment as "dual diagnosis" — true mental illness occurring with drug dependency. Rather, prolonged use of the drug decreases their capacity for self-growth and learning (Bennett, 1992). Psychologically, addicted women have higher levels of depression, anxiety, and sense of powerlessness and lower levels of self-esteem and self-confidence (Burns, Melamed, Burns, Chasnoff, & Hatcher, 1985); depression alone would put the infant-parent relationship in jeopardy. The pregnant woman who uses drugs also must deal with the sense of guilt and shame of "hurting" her growing fetus by drug use (Daghestani, 1988). The effect of the infant on the mother is intensified in the case of high-risk infancy. Whether or not the mother was emotionally unstable before the birth, a high-risk infant has the potential for destabilizing her (Burns & Burns, 1988).

Childhood sexual abuse puts women at risk for alcohol abuse, as well as for other serious adverse psychological consequences. Heavy-drinking women also are more likely to be victims of the alcohol-related sexual aggression of others. Women often date their drinking to a particular precipitating event, such as a miscarriage, stillbirth, or another event having to do with reproductive functioning.

Social Functioning

Preoccupation with a drug renders a person unable to participate in life (Bennett, 1992). Pregnant cocaine addicts suffer from the same social problems that affect other women addicts; criminality, prostitution, and vulnerability to physical abuse are primary concerns. The drug they crave is illegal, a problem the alcoholic woman does not have, and as tolerance builds, increased quantities make it more expensive.

Styles of parenting are rooted in the way one was parented. Many addicted and drug-abusing women are in families of intergenerational drug use or dysfunctional families; they reflect the parenting models they have experienced. Addicted women are likely to be single and living in unmarried cohabitation with men who are also drug users. As stated earlier, the mother's personality and parenting skill is of significant importance for the social development of the infant. A mother who is lonely and isolated from family and other social support may turn toward the infant for human comfort at a time when the infant should be the one who can seek comfort from the mother (Burns & Burns, 1988).

The stability that the pregnant woman or mother needs is the one thing she lacks most.

■□ SUMMARY

In this chapter we examined substance abuse and addiction. Although many of our questions can be answered by viewing addiction as a disease, some puzzling questions remain; for example, what accounts for first use of a drug, and why does it gain such a hold on some of us and not on others? In the following chapter we will examine our own feelings about addiction and women who use drugs. Those feelings may include anger and hostility toward women who are responsible for children affected by prenatal drug exposure. To work with the substance-abusing family, we must be honest with ourselves about our feelings.

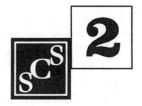

Working with the Substance-Abusing Family

As service providers, we know that children and adolescents are not separate from their families; they are always part of a family system, and our intervention with substance-exposed children must incorporate the family as much as, if not more, than with nonexposed children. As Donahue-Kilburg (1992) notes, "Nowhere is the importance of family felt more strongly than in the field of early intervention. . . . The family has become an important focus in early intervention efforts because experience and research have shown that optimal infant/toddler development can only be promoted within the family context" (p. 3). In fact, P.L. 99-457 mandates that service provision for infants and toddlers be "family centered." Furthermore, the family is regarded as a *system* because each position or role in the family is related to every other position in the family. As one member of the family changes, the whole family system changes (Kenkel, 1966). In families where the acquisition of drugs is the central focus of at least one member's existence, the family must change to cope with addiction, gain equilibrium, be rocked by another change, and struggle to cope again. It is beyond the scope of this book to discuss family systems in detail. The reader is referred to Donahue-Kilburg (1992) and Andrews and Andrews (1990) for information on family systems.

In this chapter, some questions about working with families affected by substance abuse will be addressed. Such issues are important for two reasons. First, the targets of our intervention will be not only the children affected by substance abuse but their families as well; to do otherwise would address only half the problem. Second, school personnel may know little about the drug user as a parent and about ways to channel family members into treatment for addiction problems. Some common questions are: What kind of parents are women who abuse drugs? How can I tell if a child is in a substance-abusing home, and what can I do to protect him or her? When I know that substances are abused, is there anything I can do to guide a person into treatment? Finally, when I know that a child has been substance-exposed, what should I do with the information?

◾ EFFECTS OF DRUGS ON PARENTING

Our concern with the effects of drug use is focused on impairments that have an impact on a woman's pregnancy and on her availability to enter into a predictable and nurturing relationship with her child. That relationship is crucial to our work.

Parenting, Attachment, and Communication

Studies of normal language development suggest that children build their need to communicate on interaction with a responsive caregiver, which in turn enables the child to develop an internal working model of a human relationship. A baby forms a life-long impression that he or she is emotionally attached to one or more specific persons who make him or her feel comfortable and important; that in their presence he or she can safely explore, enjoy, and profit from experiences; and that to their presence he or she must return whenever frustrated or in trouble. Thus the development of trust — the message of what can be expected of the adults in one's world — is shaped by caregiving and can be discerned very early in a child's behavior. We know that such a secure child has a good chance of entering school ready to learn, to tolerate frustration, and to look for help from the teacher when the task becomes too difficult (Shaffer, 1991).

Shaffer (1991) provides three models of human relationships that result from failure to develop this sense of security from caregiving that can be discerned in a baby's behavior by 12 to 18 months of age. (For more about attachment problems in children exposed to cocaine, see Chapter 3.)

◼️ *Ambivalence.* Ambivalent infants seem to possess the inner hunch that other people possess what they need, but will part with it with great reluctance, perhaps only if tricked or forced. The basic message these babies give to their caregivers is, "I need you with me at all times, but I am never content with what you offer me."

◼️ *Avoidance.* Avoidance babies appear quite independent, for they have acquired the belief that it is never safe to explore anything new or challenging in the presence of another person, and that the best way to live is to do everything alone. The basic message they give to their caregivers is "I don't need you; please leave me alone."

◼️ *Emptiness.* The empty infant has the belief that no one is special, that all human partners are interchangeable because they are all equally insignificant. Infants who feel emptiness often fall victim to a range of early disturbances: failure to thrive, sleep disorders, and head-banging. They appear depressed or even retarded.

All three groups arrive at school with approximately the same range of native intelligence as their more secure counterparts, but with very different strategies for learning. The ambivalent babies reach the primary grades with a very low tolerance for frustration. Their way of asking for help is to grow whiny or throw a tantrum. Teachers see them as helpless and tend to overprotect them. The avoidant babies also reach school with a low tolerance for frustration, but they are more aggressive and tend to single out ambivalent kids as their prey. Their manner of relating to teachers is often provocative. Some teachers react to this with irritation and dislike; others respond by becoming detached. Either reaction tends to further reinforce the children's avoidant stance. The empty children enter school exhibiting bizarre behaviors. They are often seen as retarded and tend to become consumers of our vast array of special services (Shaffer, 1991).

When the caregiver is dependent on a drug, the care the baby receives over the first few months of life is unpredictable. The care may diminish until it becomes nonexistent. Burns and Burns (1988) report anecdotal accounts by mothers who use drugs that relate their inability to make themselves get out of bed in the morning to care for their crying babies. Their feeding practices show little sensitivity to the needs of the infant. Attempts to interact with toys often find the play directed toward the mother's needs rather than those of her child. These mothers are described as immature women who demonstrate an abnormal degree of egocentrism in the way they go about parenting. They frequently view the birth of the child as a gift for themselves and continue to interpret the child's growth and development in terms of their own needs. In addition, it is not unusual for drug-dependent mothers to admit to child abuse, even in such a way that it seems that they are oblivious to the seriousness of the abuse (Burns & Burns, 1988).

Mothers' behaviors that are important to us as school service providers are described as follows (Burns & Burns, 1988):

> They have a great deal of difficulty understanding their infants' communications, since these communications are at first mostly expressions of the child's needs rather than responses to the mother's neediness. These mothers interpret their infant's attempts to communicate as demanding and inappropriate; and consequently they reject or criticize these early efforts to interact. At a time when their infant desperately needs encouragement to persist in social interaction, a message of discouragement is encountered instead. Parenting is experienced by the infant as a negative influence, as though the infants' growth and development were in competition with or at the expense of the mother's welfare. (p. 162)

Furthermore, when we consider that the infant may also be affected by the drug abuse prenatally and that both the infant and the principal caregiver come to the dyad at high risk for dysfunction in their interactions, the risk for dysfunction grows exponentially and the prognosis for recovery is likewise diminished.

An experience of mine when I worked as a home visitor with the county Department of Public Health may serve as an example of unpredictability and loss of trust in a child at risk for a communication disorder. The public health nurse and I arrived at a home at 11:00 A.M., the time agreed on at our last visit to this home the previous week, to visit Connie and her two children, Marilyn 2 years old and David 8 months old. They were clients in a program for at-risk infant outcome in which they were to be visited at least weekly while the baby — David — was under 1 year old. Twenty-six year old Connie was considered at risk for neglect due to her abuse of alcohol. Four older children had been removed from her care, and we were hopeful that she could learn to parent these younger ones. Repeated loud knocks at the door brought Marilyn, wearing only a tee-shirt, who let us in. We called to Connie who was upstairs and she appeared holding a soaking wet David. The previous night's party was evident; bottles were everywhere, along with discarded plates of food. Connie said she did not remember that we were coming that day. As we talked, Marilyn began to eat some cold spaghetti that was left on a plate. I suggested that we would be glad to wait while she fixed breakfast for the children. Connie said that the children were not hungry, and they would all just like to go back to bed as soon as we left. Soon after that visit Marilyn and David were removed from Connie by social services (not as a result of our visit) and placed in a foster home where I continued to visit David. I had identified him as significantly at risk for communication problems from his scores on the Early Language Milestones Screening Scale (Coplan, 1984). His foster mother had several other children in her home besides David and Marilyn. She was diligent about keeping the children well-fed, dry, and on schedule. She reported that David had cried the first few nights with her, but she had not responded and he then slept through the night. I spent 2 hours per week with David for the next few months. My main goal was for him to smile, but I did not succeed; the look of anxiety — the same look he had when he was with his mother — never left his face. He responded with some interest to the toys and pictures I brought, but his only sounds during that time were short vowel sounds that could best be categorized as whimpers. David did not trust me anymore than he trusted the other adults in his world, and I was not going to change his perception by dropping into his life a couple of times a week. I suspect that the behavior I observed was indicative of Shaffer's (1991) model of emptiness that will become evident in David's school performance later.

Fathers and Other Family Members

Thus far we have discussed the infant's caregiver as if the mother were single and without support, and that is true in the majority of cases (Burns & Burns, 1988). However, families can include families of origin in which the birth mother is not involved with the child, foster care families, and adoptive families. In the former, the father or grandparents may raise the child, perhaps with the hope that an addicted mother will come back to them.

We must be prepared to relate to caregivers other than the mother in our treatment of the child. When the family is intact and the mother's drug use is the only problem, an enormous burden may be shifted to the father. Only if he is a special person will he be able to bear such a burden.

A case in point, described in Chapter 6, is Melinda's father. Everyone involved in Melinda's care, myself included, regarded her father's influence and interference with our advice as "not normal." In retrospect, however, I must agree with Allred (1992) who stressed that professionals should suspend judgment regarding the normalcy of spousal roles in dysfunctional families because there is little consensus on what is normal, and what is viewed as dysfunctional in such families may actually be adaptive. Melinda's father took over her care and did the best he could with his resources.

Grandparents or even great-grandparents may be the family members who assume responsibility for the children of their addicted children. A group of grandparents in East Oakland, California, has formed a group called Grandparents as Second Parents (GASP, 1992) for mutual support. A young grandmother who had taken in four of her daughter's children, and who has the two youngest of her own six children still at home, said:

> All I can say is, Lord help me to cope. I'm running to the school and running to the hospital all the time. . . . I'm like a robot. . . . I'm really hurting. My own two kids say, When are they going home and I say, They're not going anyplace — they are home. . . . I pray to God that I can hang in there 'cause I'm really tired and I'm really hurting.

Another member, a great-grandmother, said:

> I'm really, really angry. I've tried everything with my granddaughter since 1981. I thought maybe if I put in for legal guardian for the children it would make her straighten up, but it didn't. . . . For so long I thought I was the only one. My great-grandson can show me every drug house from Sacramento to Oakland. She keeps telling him she's going to do something and then she don't do it. Like for his birthday she said she was going to take him to the Ice Capades. I knew she wouldn't show up. We sat there the whole evening hugging each other and she didn't show up.

The GASP group serves as an advocacy group; these grandparents feel at a disadvantage because they do not have the financial support of the state as do foster parents. They believe that a very important function of GASP is to serve as an information and referral system. They have established what they call a "warm line" for other grandparents throughout the country (see Appendix B, second listing). As one grandmother put it, "We want it to feel like a warm fuzzy — like someone is hugging them when they call."

■❏ GUIDELINES FOR WORKING WITH FAMILIES

The ideal model for family intervention is a community-based comprehensive program (described in Chapter 4) in which a mother receives treatment for her addiction while her children receive early intervention. That model is not found in our public schools, however. The following guidelines are for school personnel who have the advantage of working with a multidisciplinary or transdisciplinary team so that the family is at least minimally involved with school or intervention services for the child.

■ Use the Individualized Family Service Plan (IFSP) model with the collaboration of as many services as possible (Bennett, 1992); the intervention team in collaboration with other community service agencies and a service coordinator is ideal. This translates clinically into "beginning where the family is" (Trout & Foley, 1989). For example, the most appropriate suggestions for improving communication between a mother and child by establishing consistency and predictability become unrealistic if the mother is homeless or lives in a situation where others intrude on her parenting. Goals for the IFSP would then become establishing a safe, secure environment that enables the mother to attend to her child.

■ Help the family to participate in goal setting, choose options for interventions, and take responsibility for needs and problems in ways that are consistent with the child's needs.

■ Help the family to experience immediate success in solving a problem or meeting a need. Use their strengths for solving small problems first and increase their faith in themselves (Bennett, 1992).

■ Help the family to develop new behaviors and skills that decrease the need for help in order to promote independence.

■ Help the family to see improvement in their condition and to see themselves as responsible for the change.

■❏ INTERVENTION ISSUES

When we speak about intervention, it should be made very clear that school personnel are not expected to treat parents' addictions. That is a process best left to experts in the field of substance abuse. The mother's recovery treatment and barriers to treatment for women addicted to drugs are discussed in Chapter 7.

Why, then, are we concerned with treatment for the mother when we are treating her child? What difference does it make whether the mother is using, sober, in early recovery, or recovering? As previously suggested, treatment of the child must consider the family unit as a whole. Crites, Fischer, McNeish-Stengel, and Siegel (1992) give several reasons why substance abuse treatment for a child's family is crucial to our treatment of the child.

First, there is an implicit threat that a child may be removed from the home if drugs are used and if the mother is not in some phase of treatment. The prevailing attitude among child professionals is that children should remain in the home, if at all possible, for a number of reasons, not the least of which is the difficulty in finding good foster care. Second, as has been stated previously, families for whom obtaining drugs is the most important thing in life cannot be nurturing families for young children. It has been demonstrated that substance abuse treatment for the mother does make a difference in the social and developmental capacity of her children. Finally, early intervention depends on helping parents, and addicted parents are not amenable to such help by a school provider.

So if we must be concerned about the caregiver's sobriety or lack of it, what should we do? We should be able to recognize substance abuse, we should know how to open up the issues with a parent, we should be able to make an intelligent referral, and we should be aware of the special problems the mother will face during recovery. The following sections rely heavily on the work of Schafer (1989) who wrote from his professional experience as a psychologist and infant mental health worker.

Recognizing Substance Abuse

Cocaine

It is important to remember that all of the following signs are ambiguous. A chronically runny nose can signify cocaine abuse, since snorting coke damages the mucous tissue of the nasal passages; but a runny nose may also indicate a chronic allergy. In general, cocaine addicts are likely to be underweight. They often complain of headaches, insomnia, exhaustion, and may have a chronically runny nose. When high, they are talkative, look restless, excited, "motor running fast," and have dilated pupils. You may be able to actually see a racing pulse if you look closely at a prominent artery. When down, they look exhausted, as though they had not slept well. They tend to be silent, depressed, perhaps even suicidal. A woman who behaves one way on some visits and another way at other times may simply be exhibiting the up and down phases of her addiction.

Alcohol

Alcohol abuse is both easier and harder to spot. Think back to the alcoholic you were asked to picture at the beginning of this book. Perhaps you smelled alcohol on the clothes or breath. (If you smell alcohol and the person has not had a drink that day, you are smelling it on clothing, and that probably indicates heavy and frequent drinking.) We can also recognize fairly easily the slurred speech, unsteady gait, slowed reflexes, and glazed eyes of current intoxication. But it is more difficult to pick up the telltale signs of a weekend or episodic binge drinker. Some clues which *may* indicate an alcohol problem are a general feeling of disorganization about their lives, a noticeable blurriness of memory about events, or an inability to explain why and how major events in one's life occurred. Other signs may be a series of personal or professional losses, none of which seem to have obvious causes. Thus, a person who has lost several spouses, friendships, or jobs, and has little idea why, may be a chronic heavy drinker (Schafer, 1989).

Discovering Substance Abuse

How can we as providers or child-finders talk to parents about their substance abuse? It might be well to reflect on why we feel we need to ask. After all, we do not ponder long to find the appropriate words with which to enquire about birth history, early accidents, or language development. Yet, when it comes to drugs, we hesitate because we have our own feelings about drug use. In Chapter 5, I discuss my own experience with students when viewing a tape of the optimum way to take an alcohol history and go on to conclude that for those who find taking a drinking history too difficult, referral to a genetics clinic is the best option. Shafer (1989) believes that most of us have a secret belief that addiction is basically a fundamental weakness, but a weakness of a very special kind; it is a weakness which the addicted *should* be able to control. (Indeed, treatment programs have control as a basic premise, with 12-step programs being the best example.) This belief, and the contradiction contained in it, can make us subtly magnify the addict's defeat while we simultaneously blame her for her condition. This is probably even more likely when the addict happens to be a mother. In the back of our minds there is a feeling of horror: "How could you *do* this to your baby?" Now, if you just said to yourself, "No, I don't feel that way," be careful. Quite often, the first clue we have that we are struggling with our own inner anger, denial, and disapproval is the discomfort we feel over asking the obvious questions (Schafer, 1989).

Schafer (1989) draws the analogy of addiction being like a relationship — like being in love.

> You are introduced, there is a magic, a chemistry if you will; you begin to invest more and more of your time and energy thinking about making plans with and enjoying the presence of the beloved. You stop seeing friends as much, your family relationships suffer, perhaps your job as well. But nothing seems to matter as much as being with that someone who makes you feel so wonderful. Now, the reality may be that you've fallen in love with someone who constantly betrays you behind your back. But how do you feel about the friend who comes up to you with the bad news? If you've ever been in such a relationship, or had a close friend go through the experience, you know firsthand just how delicate a moment it is. And that's what we are faced with when we are talking with somebody in denial. This is their love we are discussing. If we want to help, we need to be respectful of that love, of the desire for happiness from which it arose, for the joy it succeeded in bringing. When we inquire about drug use, the frame of mind we would ideally like to have is simply this: "Tell me about your friend Cocaine; how does it feel to be with him?" If we can just keep that frame of mind, then it is really no great trick to find the proper words to ask the next important questions: "When did you meet him? Who introduced you? What did you think of him the first time? How often do you go out together now? What do you do? How did he treat you at first, and how does he treat you now?" In short, one can take the history of a drug addiction just like one takes the history of a love relationship. What one says at the end of such a history may simply be: "You've given up a lot for this love haven't you? It must be very important to you". (p. 3)

Assessing Substance Abuse

It would be naive to expect that talking to a substance-using mother and drawing her out in such a manner could happen in an intake visit. Would any of us want to discuss our love relationships with a stranger? If it happens at all, it is most likely in a trusting relationship built up over six to eight visits — the kind of relationship that a home visitor can build, although it should not be ruled out in a school or early intervention program where the provider and mother have time together. Whether or not that kind of relationship is built, substance abuse professionals have devised some general rules that we should be able to incorporate in our history-taking and other encounters with caregivers (Schafer, 1989):

- Any time a parent mentions drug use, whether by herself or by others, do not let it drop without showing some interest. If she mentions a family member who uses, you can ask how and when he began, what changes she has seen in him, and so forth; then you can ask who else in the family uses. You will have learned something valuable. But if you show no interest, you will give her the powerful message that you do not want to know.
- Do not ask questions that can be answered by yes or no. We know this rule from our training in interviewing techniques, but it is particularly cogent here. For example, in asking about a family member, it is better not to ask, "Do other members of your family use?" Such a question is easily answered negatively. It is much better to ask, "Who else in your family uses crack?"
- Be specific. Do not just ask about drugs, ask about coke, crack, pot, alcohol, uppers, and downers.

Referral for Treatment

Let us assume that the mother has now let you know that she has a substance problem. She probably will be ambivalent about seeking help. When she says that she is ready to work on her problem, seize the moment. Be ready with a phone number and help her make the call. You will need to do some previous homework by making inquiries into treatment facilities in your community. You may talk it over with your early intervention team, if you have one, or with the high school guidance counselor who must deal with student substance abuse problems and who will probably know about treatment programs. Another source is the yellow pages of the phone book. If your client does not have the resources for a private treatment facility, call them anyway and ask where in the community they refer those who cannot pay. If these sources do not yield a treatment program, try the city or county health department. If you are caught without a referral program when the opening comes, tell her you will find out and then follow up at the earliest opportunity. Her resolve may melt away when time elapses.

Recovery and Relapse

This section deals with special problems of working with a child whose mother is in early recovery — the first 12 to 24 months of sobriety. Since we are working with the principle that the mother and child are in a family system, and that what happens with the mother has a direct effect on the child, the mother's success in recovery has an influence on our ability to make changes and carry out our goals.

The first question is whether the mother is actually in recovery (Schafer, 1990). Just because she has been through a recovery program does not assure sobriety. Many women and men go through treatment many times before they can maintain sobriety. Suppose the following: The mother is simply unable to utilize any of your suggestions. The suggestions require far too much self-control, patience, and calm. Your words seem to simply fall on deaf ears. The recovering mother will usually be fairly vulnerable, but she should be able to hear some of what you say and to follow through with part of it. If she seems to you to be simply unable to follow through at all, you may want to ask yourself if you are dealing with a mother who is actively using. If so, your work to help her with her child's needs will most certainly fail because she simply cannot hear you. The drug is more powerful than either you or her child. Your only options are to go back to helping her find treatment or to stop trying to have her involved with your work (Schafer, 1990).

Guidelines for Working with Recovery

Expect Relapse to Occur

Treatment experts have learned to take relapse in stride. It does not mean that sobriety will not eventually be accomplished. While relapse is occurring, the mother will experience enormous discouragement and disappointment. Do not be afraid to say that you think she is having trouble working on her program and encourage her to go back to it. There are many stories of women who kicked their drug habits and became successful parents. Burns and Burns (1988) hypothesize that it is plausible to believe that the process of getting and maintaining sobriety brings about other changes as well, such as maturity, self-esteem, and the ability to see beyond one's own needs, that in turn aid parenting. Remember, if a mother is actively using, she cannot hear you and you cannot count on her. If she is in recovery, you have a chance. The rewards can be great.

The Goals of Recovery May Conflict
with Therapy Goals for the Child

The mother is focused on her own needs and keeping herself sober; she may also have a counselor who sees the mother's needs as paramount. My own experience may serve as an example. I was an advisor to a project aimed at enhancing the skills of mothers and caregivers to foster the development of language and preliteracy skills in young children. One of the several centers where caregiver training was given was a center for mothers recovering from crack addiction and their children. The other centers were child-centered; this one was mother-centered. A main goal of treatment for the mothers was to have them take responsibility for their children's care. In one instance, the project staff recommended a hearing test for a child who showed symptoms of hearing loss. The test could be given at the clinic across the street from the center. The project staff person arranged the appointment and would have taken the mother and child to the appointment, except that the center staff would not allow it. Their goal was to have the child's mother follow through by taking the child herself. When the mother did not follow through, the child did not get the hearing test. It is easy for us to empathize with the frustration of the project staff: a child who needed a service went without it. But the center staff did not feel that they should relieve the mother of her responsibility and the consequences of not accepting that responsibilty.

Keep the Mother Very Tightly Focused

She will be trying hard to stay sober, and she needs success to celebrate in her recovery and in the work both of you do with her child. When she carries out her assignment with you, seize on how well she did and praise her.

Do Not Expect Too Much

Relapse and failure are hard on providers, and it is easy to give up. Expect more broken appointments and noncompliance than with any other families you have worked with. Remember that making plans, even for the next day, is not a priority for this mother. If you let it make you angry, you will be ineffective. We cannot expect to change patterns that have been in place for years in a few weeks or months. Nor can we change underlying social causes. However, there have been cases where an individual provider has been the only person a mother trusted and that trust allowed her to be open to change. Choose realistic goals in the IFSP process and work toward them.

Collaborate

These families require the services of every member of the team, especially the service coordinator and social worker. Professional burn-out is accelerated when the provider works with substance abuse. Keep your personal reinforcement and networking systems active and working: from supervisors, other providers, school personnel, and outside professionals. Share frustrations and ideas.

Be Careful

My whole philosophy has been to work with the child as part of a dyad and family system, and my experience of many years as a home-visitor has only strengthened that conviction. I strongly believe that home visits are an important part of early intervention and they should be made whenever possible. As a speech-language pathologist for Head Start in the 1970s, I went into neighborhoods where the crime rates were high. Carrying my orange Peabody Language kit, I was sure that I was watched, but I did not feel threatened, nor did anything ever happen to me. But that was before the crack epidemic of the 1980s when streets became really dangerous. You need not go anywhere that you do not feel safe. If you go to neighborhoods and homes where there is drug use and dealing, do not go alone and reserve the right to leave abruptly. I do not give out my home phone number under any circumstances to drug-using clients. The number that I give them is an office phone with an answering machine; they know that I will return the call promptly.

Watch for Signs of Abuse and Neglect

When a dependent child is at high risk for neglect and abuse in a certain environment, a referral to children's protective services is necessary. Proper steps may have to be taken to have the child removed from such situations. The more this can be accomplished in a supportive nonthreatening atmosphere, the greater will be the likelihood that the mother can be rehabilitated and the family environment improved for the welfare of mother and child. For many mothers, the desire to nurture children can be a powerful motivation for sobriety. Yet termination of maternal rights must be a consideration in situations where sobriety cannot be achieved and the children continue to be neglected or abused (Streissguth & Giunta, 1988).

■❏ LABELING

The final topic in this chapter concerns what providers should do with the information that a child has been substance-exposed. Perhaps the most important principle to keep in mind is that the needs of the child come first. Such a statement surely does not appear to be in conflict with our professional standards. We chose our profession because we wanted to serve children and adults who need our help and expertise. But how can we serve children best? Should they always be *labeled* as children whose problems stem from drug abuse? If the child is receiving intervention, does it really matter that the etiology is identified as drug-related? If a child is identified as having an alcohol-related disorder, must we do anything other than put that child in our caseload and use appropriate intervention for the problem? As previously mentioned, the IFSP model is recommended for intervention, so it is likely that the information will be shared, at least with the IFSP team. But what about passing the information along? What about devoting special classrooms to substance-exposed children?

Labeling for Alcohol-Related Problems

Throughout this book, references are made to lack of data; FAS in particular is difficult to identify at birth and is likely to be overlooked by physicians. For purposes of data collection, it is imperative that we document alcohol-related disorders as risk factors in school records when we know they are present, if we are to ever gain an understanding of efficacy in treatment programs for alcohol-related disorders. But what about labeling the child? Is that not in conflict with the statment made earlier that the needs of the child come first? There is no reason to think that the child will not be well served if labeled as having an alcohol-related etiology. In fact, evidence suggests that the children, their foster parents, and even their biologic mothers are often relieved to find out there is a known cause for their difficulties with learning and communication (Dorris, 1989). Furthermore, treatment can then proceed along the lines known to be most efficacious for children with alcohol-related problems. Diagnosis of FAS is a medical diagnosis; procedures for obtaining that diagnosis are given in Chapter 5. It is important for the child, the teacher, the provider, and for the research community that the diagnosis is made. To treat the child *as if* the diagnosis were made, but not take steps to get the diagnosis confirmed because that is the easiest path, does not serve anyone well. Documented cases of FAS should receive early intervention under P.L. 99-457 guidelines (see Chapter 8).

Labeling for Cocaine-Related Problems

Affixing a cocaine- or crack-induced etiology to a child is more problematic than documenting an alcohol etiology for a number of reasons, not the least of which is the constantly shifting legal and political climate surrounding the use of illegal substances. Crack-exposed children are more easily identified at birth than alcohol-exposed children due to toxicology screens that are becoming routine in many hospitals. Even so, the majority of cases of maternal substance abuse in pregnancy go undetected and unreported (Chasnoff, 1988). In some communities, a positive screen means that the baby will be removed from the mother until the mother proves that she is in recovery; in others the courts and the foster care system are too overwhelmed to remove these babies. In any case, the label will most likely be given at birth, usually before any interventionist sees the child. There is no assurance, however, that the label will follow the child when he or she enters school. Rivers and Hedrick (1992) found from a survey of speech-language pathologists that clinical reports about a given child as the product of a cocaine pregnancy were not always retained or made available to schools or health care providers. The authors concluded that clinicians should acquire in-depth history data themselves and not rely on reports that accompany the child. Certainly, we must be aware that the absence of data on drug exposure does not mean a child was not exposed. Exposure to cocaine may or may not produce sequelae, and the adverse effects are most often seen in children who are not only exposed to cocaine but also are premature, of low birth weight, and sick; many other children may have been exposed, but because they were of normal birth weight and there was no suspicion of drug use, they did not receive a toxicology screen at birth. For such children, the expectation of problems may indeed be unrealistic; at this time we simply do not know. A drug-related disability should be known by all who work with a child who shows difficulties; the label is not warranted, however, for children who do not appear to be affected by the drug exposure. Some children exposed to cocaine will show symptoms; others may be free of symptoms. The problem is that professionals may use a child's drug exposure to account for any and all problems that appear when that need not be the case. The stigma of "crack kid" has caused needless harm and pain to many children. For those reasons, labeling a child as drug exposed in the absence of symptoms does not serve the child well.

In summary, if a child is suspected of having an alcohol-related disorder, every effort should be made to get a diagnosis and document it in the child's school record. If, in obtaining a history, drug use is mentioned, it should, of course, be recorded. However, the label of "crack kid" is so highly stigmatizing, and we have so little information about long-term outcome, that, in the absence of symptoms, the child is better served to not be labeled by each succeeding provider as he or she passes through the school system.

■□ SUMMARY

In this chapter, guidelines for working with the substance-using family have been given. All of us who work with affected families must look at our own attitudes concerning substance abuse and examine our own anger at behaviors that affect unborn children before we can work effectively with these families. In the following chapters, behaviors of children exposed prenatally to drugs will be examined and suggestions will be given for intervention in a school setting.

Prenatal Cocaine Exposure

A rapidly growing body of research strongly suggests that prenatal substance exposure is linked to health problems in the newborn as well as to problems in the child's development (Zuckerman, 1991). Although media attention has focused primarily on crack cocaine use by pregnant women, that examination ignores the thousands of pregnant women who use and abuse one or more other legal and illegal drugs. We tend to think of the legal drugs, alcohol and nicotine, as the "good drugs" and illegal drugs, such as cocaine, heroin, and PCP, as the "bad drugs," although prenatal exposure to alcohol and nicotine have more deleterious effects on the fetus than the "bad drugs."

The polydrug nature of most substance use makes it exceptionally difficult to determine the effects of any one drug on subsequent child development. The prenatally exposed babies cited in most of the research in this chapter are not really "crack" or "cocaine" babies but rather "polydrug" babies. It is impossible to say which of the effects, often misattributed to cocaine alone in the popular press, are actually due to cocaine, which to other substances used, and which to the combination. Nevertheless, based on what we know about child development in general, the deficits that some drug-exposed infants and toddlers exhibit may predict subsequent developmental problems. Other findings from developmental literature indicate that even children who are impaired by exposure to drugs in utero can and should be helped by concerted early intervention programs (Kronstadt, 1991).

Articles in the popular press tell of the "lost generation" of children "addicted" to crack cocaine. Media coverage has typically focused on worst case scenarios. The nation's schools are warned to get ready for the onslaught of the wave of crack children that is now headed for them. The following article (Rist, 1990) aimed at school board members is an example of perpetration of fears that are unwarranted:

> The first wave of crack babies — born after crack cocaine hit the streets in 1985 — could be enrolling in your kindergarten classes next fall.
>
> The arrival of those first afflicted youngsters will mark the beginning of a struggle that will leave your resources depleted and your compassion tested. And just about your only chance of being equal to the task is to appreciate it now and begin at once to prepare your schools. This is something new — and bad.
>
> Here's how one psychologist describes the growing number of children prenatally exposed to crack cocaine: They're kids wired for 110 volts, living in a 220-volt world. And according to available evidence, many of these children will not be easy to talk to — let alone teach.
>
> What cocaine-exposed newborns go through during the days and weeks after birth offers a bad enough start on life: Some have birth defects — deformed hearts, lungs, digestive systems, or limbs — attributed to cocaine exposure in the uterus. Most are small and underweight. Nearly all are irritable, tremulous, and difficult to soothe for at least the first three months. Worse, many evidently suffer permanent neurological damage from prenatal drug exposure. For them, coping with the normal activities and stimuli of daily life will be difficult.
>
> . . . Douglas Besharov, former director of the National Center on Child Abuse and currently a scholar at the American Enterprise Institute, has dubbed these kids a potential "bio-underclass" — a cohort of children whose combined physiological damage and extreme socioeconomic disadvantage could foredoom them to a life of inferiority.
>
> . . . Although, at first glance, drug-exposed children might not look much different from other youngsters, the long-term effects of fetal drug exposure emerge as the children begin interacting in the larger world. In the typical classroom environment — where noises, voices, instructions, questions, interactions, and distractions crowd one upon the other — cocaine-exposed children tend to react in one of two ways. They withdraw completely, or they become wild and difficult to control.
>
> Like 110-volt fuses when a burst of current pulses through and overloads them, these children are prone to short-circuit or burn out with too much stimulation. How your schools get ready to handle them — how you prepare to make this growing population of innocent victims the best they can be — is the question facing your school board right now. (p. 19)

This article is not unusual in its sense of urgency and alarm. However, in getting the attention of school boards and asking them to prepare for a wave of children like none we have ever seen before, some damaging myths are perpetuated that do not stand up to scrutiny.

The first myth is that all children exposed to cocaine will experience adverse effects. In fact, most of the children exposed to drugs prenatally are not adversely affected. In most studies of cocaine use in pregnancy, less than half of the cocaine-exposed neonates demonstrated effects of intrauterine cocaine exposure: low birth weight, prematurity, intrauterine growth retardation, small head circumference, and neurobehavioral deficits (Chasnoff, Griffith, MacGregor, Dirkes, & Burns, 1989; Little, Snell, Klein, & Gilstrap, 1989). According to Mayes, Granger, Borstein, and Zuckerman (1991):

> Predictions of an adverse developmental outcome for these children are being made despite a lack of supportive scientific evidence. Whatever the true outcome, we are concerned that premature conclusions about the severity and universality of cocaine effects are in themselves potentially harmful to children. (p. 406)

The second myth is that "these children" require unprecedented resources. This prediction presumes that effective early intervention practices used for other high-risk preschoolers will not be adequate for drug-exposed children and that all school-age children affected by drug exposure will have to be served in special education programs (Rinkel, 1992). There is no doubt that children exposed prenatally to drugs pose serious challenges to school personnel. We know that prenatal exposure to cocaine constitutes a *risk* for development in many areas. But the direct effects of the drug may not be the sole cause of a child's problem, nor is it irreversible. The important point is that there is no typical cocaine-exposed child. In fact, according to Kronstadt (1991), in many ways, prenatally drug-exposed children look much like other children who live in similarly chaotic homes or neighborhoods. Adverse effects may or may not be present, if present, they may occur in a continuum of severity, and may be ameliorated.

The third myth is the inevitability of doom. "Biologic underclass" connotes a permanent condition for a class of people — the labelling of a generation. As we shall see from the incidence studies discussed later in this chapter, more white women take drugs, including cocaine, than black or Hispanic women. Just as many women test positive for cocaine in private hospitals as in public hospitals, and there are as many drugs in the rural areas of the United States as in the inner cities. Furthermore, early intervention works and is even more promising for children exposed to cocaine than it is for children prenatally exposed to alcohol.

In this chapter, the following questions will be addressed: How do we know if a child has been exposed to drugs? How common is prenatal exposure? What happens to the mother when she uses cocaine? To the fetus? Does prenatal exposure to cocaine mean there are predictable patterns of development? What are the expected deleterious effects of prenatal cocaine exposure? How long do they last? What are the direct and indirect effects of prenatal cocaine exposure? The effects of cocaine will be viewed within a conceptual framework, and some background on cocaine will be presented.

Historical Perspective

Cocaine is extracted from the leaf of a small tree known as the coca, which is native to South America. It's medical use as an anesthetic was discovered in 1884. Before that time it was widely used in various tonics and "pick-me-ups," including Coca-Cola. In 1914 it was restricted by the Harrison Narcotic Act, which effectively drove it underground. Cocaine is in no way a narcotic and is very dissimilar from opiates and alcohol, both pharmacologically and behaviorally. During the 1960s cocaine use began to increase for reasons that had much to do with the attitudes of middle class young people and growth of the entire drug culture (McKim, 1991).

◼◻ INCIDENCE

Identification of Cocaine Exposure

Before we discuss the incidence of prenatal cocaine exposure, it is important to understand how the statistics are compiled, that is, how cocaine use during pregnancy is identified. There are two ways to identify prenatal drug use: questions and laboratory assessments. Both are problematic with unreliable results.

Questions

According to estimates from the 1990 National Household Survey (National Institute on Drug Abuse, 1991), over 6 million Americans admitted to cocaine use in the year prior to the survey. The survey did not ask about pregnancy, only ages of respondents. Of women in the child-bearing age group of 18 to 25 years old, 22.2% of white, 21.2% of black, and 15.4% of Hispanic women said they had used illegal drugs in the past year. In the age group of 12 to 17 years old, 15% of white, 8% of black, and 11.1% of Hispanic women had used drugs. Gomby and Shiono (1991) have estimated that 554,400 to 739,200 infants each year may be exposed in utero to one or more illicit drugs. The true figures are probably much higher; the Household Survey samples only households (which excludes the homeless and those living in penal institutions) with a telephone. It also assumes that drug users will actually admit an illegal activity to a stranger who is identified as working for the U.S. government. Even so, the numbers reflect an abuse problem of epidemic proportions (McNagy & Parker, 1992). An important finding of the Household Survey, however, is that illegal drug use is not just a problem of black women in the inner cities; more whites than minorities use drugs and they are located in rural and suburban America.

Laboratory Assessments

Unlike alcohol, cocaine use can be detected by screening at birth through urine toxicological analysis for a metabolite of cocaine called benzoylecgonine. A positive screen for either the mother or the neonate means that the mother used cocaine within approximately the previous 48 hours, but it does not uncover cocaine use prior to that time. Urine screens are routinely done only on suspicion of drug use in most hospitals. A more sensitive test to determine if a neonate has been exposed to any of four drugs (cocaine, heroin, marijuana, and amphetamines) during gestation is available in which a first stool specimen (known as meconium in the neonatal period) is sent to a laboratory for analysis (Ostrea, Parks, & Brady, 1989). However, neither the urine or meconium screens are completely reliable. The threshold for detection of the metabolite in urine is set by federal standards (National Institute of Drug Abuse) at 300 ng/ml. Actually, the cocaine metabolite can be detected at a lower level, 100 ng/ml, but if the concentration is below 300 ng/ml, the laboratory will call it negative (Chasnoff, 1992). Likewise, it is possible that the meconium will not be sampled correctly; the sample may not be adequate to contain enough of the drug or metabolite of the drug to show up in the test results. The newest method of detection is through hair samples. The hair of the mother or baby not only discloses cocaine use, but also shows a temporal pattern of use throughout the shaft of the hair. However, this test also has drawbacks: Bleaching the hair will change its composition and cutting it destroys the evidence. Furthermore, there is a racial difference in the way hair retains cocaine. Black and coarse hair retains the drug longer than blond and fine hair, thus there is a risk of racially biased results (Chasnoff, 1992).

Perhaps the best method of drug use detection is careful, and time-consuming history-taking. A woman who takes illegal drugs is unlikely to admit it to someone whom she does not trust when she knows or suspects that admission is more likely to bring about punishment than help.

State of Incidence Knowledge

At present, no reliable national estimates of the extent or patterns of cocaine use during pregnancy exist. Depending on the methods used and the populations studied, prevalence estimates from individual hospitals range from 3% to 50% of live births. The higher estimates are most often reported from centers serving poor, inner city mothers (Mayes, Granger, Bornstein, & Zuckerman, 1991).

There is no consensus on the percentage of infants exposed because, as discussed above, the testing methods and the criteria for women chosen to be tested vary widely. Some hospitals do not have a protocol for assessing drug use during pregnancy; others require testing only if the mother reported drug use or the infant manifested drug withdrawal signs (U.S. General Accounting Office Report to the Chairman, Committe on Finance, U.S. Senate, 1990). On the other hand, one urban hospital screened nearly 3,000 newborns for the presence of cocaine or heroin in the meconium, and over 40% tested positive (Randall, 1992). The U.S. General Accounting Office Report to the Chairman, Committe on Finance, U.S. Senate (1990) estimates that the rate of prenatal exposure would be close to 16% of newborns if screening and testing were uniform in all hospitals. Chasnoff, Landress, and Barrett (1990) found in their study in Pinellas County, Florida, that despite similar rates of substance abuse among black and white women, black women were tested and reported at approximately 10 times the rate for white women, and poor women were more likely than others to be reported. They concluded that the use of illicit drugs is common among pregnant women regardless of race and socioeconomic status.

Passive Exposure

An emergency department of a large urban hospital recently found cocaine metabolite in the urine of more than 5% of the toddlers and children treated there for routine pediatric complaints. The most likely route of exposure is second-hand smoke inhaled when adult caretakers use free-base or crack cocaine (Randall, 1992). The physiological and behavioral effects of chronic environmental exposure to cocaine in children are not well established. Reported cases have included transient neurological symptoms, such as drowsiness and unsteady gait, and seizures (Randall, 1992). Service providers who encounter such unexplained behaviors should suspect second-hand exposure and refer the child to the school nurse or health official.

Passive exposure may occur in breast-fed infants because cocaine is excreted in breast milk. Cocaine can be passed on to an infant in breast milk for 48 hours after the mother has used cocaine. Mothers who use cocaine must not breast feed their infants. Infants may also be victims of intentional cocaine administration as a form of child abuse (Giacoia, 1990).

Costs

For children who are affected, drug exposure is costly in dollars as well as quality of life. Neonatal hospital costs from delivery until medical clearance for discharge average $5,200 more for cocaine-exposed infants than for unexposed infants. The cost of infants remaining in the nursery while waiting for home and social evaluation or foster care placement increases the costs by more than $3,500. At the national level, these individual medical costs for drug-exposed neonates add up to about $500 million (Phibbs, Bateman, & Schwartz, 1991). These costs do not address the costs of long-term consequences for drug-exposed neonates.

The U.S. General Accounting Office Report to the Chairman, Committee on Finance, U.S. Senate (1990), delineates the potential impact of these children on social welfare and educational systems:

> Although definitive information is not yet available, many drug-exposed infants may have long-term learning and developmental deficiencies that could result in underachievement and excessive school dropout rates leading to adult illiteracy and unemployment. As increasing numbers of drug-exposed infants reach school age, the long-term detrimental effects of drug exposure will become more evident. The cost of minimizing the long-term effects of drug exposure will vary with the severity of disabilities. For example, at a pilot preschool program for mildly impaired prenatally drug-exposed children in Los Angeles, the per capita cost is estimated to be $17,000 per year. The Florida Department of Health and

Rehabilitative Services estimates that for those drug-exposed children who show significant physiologic or neurologic impairment total service costs to age 18 could be as high as $750,000. (p. 8)

■❏ COCAINE'S ACTION

To discuss the effects of prenatal cocaine exposure on a child, it is helpful to understand how cocaine affects the neurotransmitters in the user. Cocaine belongs to the classification of drugs known as psychomotor stimulants whose action is excitatory. The other major drugs in this class are amphetamines; thus cocaine and amphetamines are cross-tolerant (see Chapter 1). The user's perceived effects are said to be the same for amphetamines and cocaine (McKim, 1991).

Cocaine crosses the blood-brain barrier and is concentrated in the spleen, kidneys, and brain. The psychomotor stimulants activate the sympathetic nervous system causing an increase in heart rate and blood pressure and a dilation of blood vessels and the air passages in the lungs. Overdoses cause intense cardiovascular effects and may result in convulsions, respiratory depression, cardiac failure, and death. Cocaine prevents sleep and has been used to help an individual stay awake while studying or driving. Feelings of positive mood increase, such as "a sense of well-being," an "exhilaration," and "bubbling inside" (McKim, 1991).

Even at low doses, cocaine decreases consumption of both food and water; thus a pregnant woman who takes cocaine is very likely to cut down her nutritional intake. An insidious effect of cocaine usage is development of tolerance; with repeated administration, higher and higher doses are required to obtain the euphoric effect. After continuous long-term use of cocaine, a permanent depression in mood may arise from changes in the functioning of the monamine systems in the brain.

Cocaine sniffing, smoking, and injection can lead to an intense compulsion to continue use until the drug runs out or the user becomes exhausted. During such runs it is not unusual for vast sums to be spent on the drug. People have been known to sell their houses and cars to finance such binges. Many users report disturbing physiological and psychological symptoms as well: paranoid feelings, visual hallucinations, cravings, antisocial behavior, attention and concentration problems, blurred vision, coughing, muscle pains, dry skin, tremors, and weight loss. Many of the drug's harmful effects are indirect and arise from the user's lifestyle such as poor nutrition, aberrant sleep patterns, and exposure to infectious diseases, for example, AIDS (McKim, 1991). The lifestyle in a household where cocaine is used can hardly be called a nurturing environment for children.

■□ EFFECTS ON THE USER

User's Perception

If cocaine is injected, snorted, or smoked, it can be administered in concentrations sufficient to produce an intense feeling of euphoria called a "rush." Within a couple of minutes there is a numbing sensation called the "freeze," which is followed after 5 minutes by a feeling of exhilaration and well-being — a feeling of energy and the sensation of clear thoughts and perceptions. This lasts for 20 or 30 minutes and is followed by a mild depression called the "comedown" or "letdown." The letdown can be relieved immediately by another administration of the drug. The severity of the depression is related to the dose and the duration of the intake period. Cocaine is often taken in conjunction with other drugs.

Administration

Smoking or snorting cocaine delivers high doses to the brain quickly. It has become popular to smoke cocaine in several forms (Robinson, Personal Communication, 1991):

- Cocaine HCl ("C," coke, flake, snow, stardust) is the salt cocaine hydrochloride, an odorless, white powder that is snorted.
- Cocaine free base is extracted from cocaine HCl with organic solvents such as ether. It can be smoked with a free base pipe.
- Crack is cocaine mixed with a solution of baking soda. The water is evaporated, leaving crystalline chunks or "rocks" that are heated and the vapors are inhaled.

Effects on Physiology and Behavior in the User

Neurotransmitters

For the individual who uses cocaine, the high, or feeling of exhilaration, is produced by its effect on the neurotransmitters. Action of the neurotransmitters in a neural synapse will be explored in some detail for the reader who wishes to understand cocaine's mechanism of action.

THE SYNAPSE. Information is transferred between neurons at synapses. Synapses occur at the end of the axon of one cell where it terminates close to the dendrites and cell body of another cell. Figure 3–1 is a

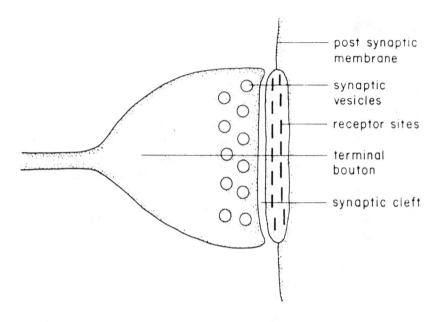

Figure 3-1
Schematic drawing of a typical synapse. From McKim, W. J. (1991).
Drugs and behavior: An introduction to behavioral pharmacology,
(2nd ed.). Englewood Cliffs, NJ: Prentice Hall, (p. 52), reproduced
with permission.

schematic drawing of a typical synapse. When the *action potential* comes
down the axon of the cell that is sending the information and it arrives at
the swelling called the terminal bouton, it causes a chemical called a
neurotransmitter to be released from the synaptic vesicles into the synaptic cleft. The neurotransmitter diffuses across the cleft, where it becomes
attached to *receptor sites.* The neurotransmitter is then reabsorbed into
the terminal bouton where it is again stored in the vesicles and recycled
(McKim, 1991).

     There are as many as 50 different neurotransmitters. Cocaine affects
the family of neurotransmitters called *monoamines* which is composed of
three *catecholamines* including dopamine, epinephrine, and norepine-
phrine. Cocaine blocks the reabsorption of the catecholamine neurotransmitter so that it stays in the cleft longer, thus producing a high
degree of stimulant and excitability (McKim, 1991).

■□ PRENATAL EXPOSURE: CONCEPTUAL FRAMEWORK

Risk vs. Deficit

Throughout this chapter, cocaine exposure will be considered a *risk* instead of the cause of deficits the child may exhibit. There is a danger in thinking about drug-exposed children in a "deficit model." A deficit model assumes that the baby has experienced some neurochemical or other fundamental damage to its capacities for self-organizing and self-righting. Symptoms of drug exposure are also observed in full-term, otherwise healthy babies who have not been exposed to drugs. However, in a deficit model, any difficulty of the drug-exposed infant is attributed to the single cause of drug exposure, and the complexities of the impact of drugs on parents and children are deemed beyond understanding and preventive interventions, even beyond professional help. The deficit model can be used to rationalize giving up on drug-exposed infants and their mothers (Weston, Ivins, Zuckerman, Jones, & Lopez, 1989).

A "risk model," on the other hand, recognizes that fetal exposure to drugs jeopardizes developmental processes but that environment may contribute to positive developmental outcomes. Prospective studies of risk have repeatedly indicated that developmental outcomes are the product of both constitutional make-up and environment. The effects of the child on the environment and the environment on the child are consistent with the transactional model of development by Samaroff and Chandler (1975) (Werner & Smith, 1982).

Direct and Indirect Effects

Perhaps the best theoretical explanation of children's individual outcomes involves *direct* and *indirect* effects of the drug that may be due to different physiological mechanisms (Jones & Lopez, 1988; Lester, et al., 1991). Direct effects include the action of cocaine on the fetus as a consequence of the transfer of the drug through the placenta. Direct effects are independent of the mother. As discussed in the section on drug action in this chapter, the fetal neurotransmitter sites are affected. This mechanism affects the sympathetic nervous system and produces vasoconstriction, an acute rise in arterial blood pressure, tachycardia, and a predisposition to ventricular arrhythmias and seizures (Cregler & Mark, 1986; Lester, 1991; Tarr & Macklin, 1987).

Indirect effects can be attributed to the fetal environment and effects on the mother's central nervous system that in turn affect the fetus (Jones & Lopez, 1988). For example, cocaine causes smooth muscle to contract, thereby precipitating preterm labor. (Cocaine is used as a method for abortion and to stimulate early labor in the belief that a small baby will be easy to deliver.) Cocaine also results in vasoconstriction of the uterine arteries and impairs the delivery of oxygen to the fetus. The mother's responses to cocaine, such as vasoconstriction, tachycardia, and increased blood pressure, all increase the chance for intermittent interruption of oxygen. The risk of abruptio placenta, in which the placenta pulls away from the uterine wall and delivers before the neonate, thus depriving the neonate of oxygen, followed by hemorrhage, shock, and anemia, is also increased (Lester et al., 1991; Tarr & Macklin, 1987), all contributing risk factors for sequelae of prematurity in the newborn.

Prenatal Environment

The theoretical linkages of direct and indirect effects can be depicted in the following diagram.

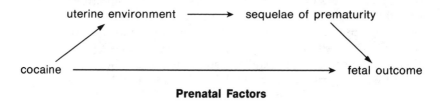

Prenatal Factors

Thus two factors influence outcome: cocaine's direct negative effect on the fetus, and cocaine's negative influence on the uterine environment which leads to the sequelae of prematurity, also affecting the outcome. Such negative factors are thought to have a *transient* effect on the infant.

For example, it is well known that the most cogent risk factor for a newborn is low birth weight. Neonates prenatally exposed to cocaine are typically of low birth weight (Chouteau, Namerow, & Leppert, 1988; Little, Snell, Klein, & Gilstrap, 1989). In a recent, and particularly well done study, McCormick, Brooks-Gunn, Workman-Daniels, Turner, and Peckham (1992), examined the range and cumulative nature of adverse health status at school age among children with lower birth weights. (Neonates exposed prenatally to cocaine were not identified as a separate group in this study.) They concluded that children born at very low birth weight experience higher rates of adverse health status at early school age across several individual dimensions of health. All low birth weight children in their study appeared to be at similar risk for "behavior problems" reported by their mothers, but lower IQ scores were concentrated among those whose birth weight was less than 1,000 grams. The authors also assessed the effect of environmental factors as reflected by maternal educational attainment. Children whose mothers had at least a high school education had higher IQs at school age; that is, the mother's education made up for the low birth weight (except for the extremely low birth weight infants), which again suggests that the risk status of low birth weight children can be ameliorated by early intervention.

Post-Natal Factors

In another diagram, we can visualize the theoretical constructs of direct and indirect environmental influences on postnatal outcome.

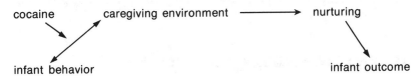

Postnatal Factors

In this diagram the influences of infant behavior and caregiving environment are depicted as an interaction with arrows going both ways. This interaction is affected by cocaine exposure on both parties to the interaction. For example, the prenatally exposed infant is fussy and hard to care for; the mother is ill equipped to deal with a fussy baby because of her own condition mediated by the drug. Thus cocaine has an indirect effect on the interaction. The caregiver is further impaired in her ability to provide nurturing, and the infant outcome is influenced negatively. These effects are considered to be *nontransient* (Lester et al., 1991).

Excitable vs. Depressed Behaviors

Lester et al. (1991) described a consensus from the research in which neurobehavioral patterns of cocaine-exposed infants can be divided into two extremes of behavior: excitable and depressed. The authors hypothesized that excitable behavior patterns are due to the direct neurotoxic effects of cocaine, and depressed behavior is due to the indirect effects of cocaine secondary to complications in the uterine environment, such as hypoxia and intrauterine growth retardation (IUGR).

Lester et al. (1991) described excitable infants as easily aroused infants who show signs such as irritability, excessive and high-pitched crying, tremors, jitteriness, and hypertonicity. Depressed behavior refers to a decrease in functional activity. Depressed infants are underaroused, are difficult to wake, and have fleeting attention and low orientation and state control scores on the Neonatal Behavior Assessment Scale (Brazelton, 1984).

Some infants may show a mixed syndrome consisting of elements of both excitable and depressed behavior, for example, infants who have a high initial threshold for reactivity and appear depressed but become very reactive when stimulated. Various combinations of excitable and depressed behavior may be observed in individual infants.

In this conceptual framework, the manifestations of prenatal cocaine exposure will be addressed as they affect the child physically and neurobehaviorally.

■□ PHYSICAL MANIFESTATIONS

Drugs taken by the mother reach the placenta via the uterine arteries. The placenta acts as a drug recipient and a drug-transferring organ. The factors that affect drug distribution in the mother will control the amount transferred to the fetus (Jones & Lopez, 1988). The action of the drug depends on its concentration at the receptor site(s). In both the woman and the fetus, distribution of the substance in the body is influenced by relative proportions of lean body mass, fat, and water and by the immaturity of the blood-brain barrier of the fetus. The drug must be metabolized by the liver and excreted by the kidneys in both mother and fetus. Drug metabolism by the fetal liver is less effective than in later life. What may not be an overdose to the mother can be an overdose to the fetus. Excretion of drugs is affected by the fact that the kidney is immature (Jones & Lopez, 1988).

Table 3–1 summarizes the physical manifestations, from direct and indirect causes, observed in infants exposed prenatally to cocaine (Fulroth, Phillips, & Durand, 1989; Hadeed & Siegel, 1989; Howard, 1989). Head circumference is the most important manifestation for long-lasting effects. According to Chasnoff, Griffith, Freier, and Murray (1992),

Table 3-1

Physical risks of prenatal cocaine exposure

Small head circumference

Low birth weight from prematurity or intrauterine growth retardation

Intrauterine cerebral and cardiac infarctions: small strokes and heart attacks

Congenital disruptions: cardiac, genitourinary, limb malformations

AIDS and other infections

---

catch-up head growth may be an important biological marker in predicting long-term development in children exposed in utero to cocaine and other drugs.

In addition, some infants have congenital anomalies as a direct result of the decrease in blood supply to the fetus. These anomalies are *disruptions,* not malformations. That is, at any time during normal fetal development, interruptions in the blood supply can result in the death of cells. For example, cocaine taken during the time that the fingers are developing can result in constriction of the blood vessels to the fingers so that the fingers suffer an *infarction:* The cells in the fingers die, and the fingers fail to develop or they drop off. Infarctions that are even more dangerous involve the infant's vascular system, causing stroke and heart attack in utero (Chasnoff, 1992). Infants born to women who use cocaine are also at risk for AIDS because the women have a high incidence of AIDS.

■□ NEUROBEHAVIORAL MANIFESTATIONS

According to Lester et al. (1991), no clear and consistent findings concerning neurobehavioral effects have been established, the news media notwithstanding. A number of studies have noted that drug-exposed infants have difficulty with state control (Anday, Cohen, Kelley, & Leitner, 1989; Chasnoff, Lewis, Griffith, & Wiley, 1989; Hume, O'Donnell, Stanger, Killam, & Gingras, 1989). Such infants are reported to: (a) be fussy and inconsolable, (b) lose state control when stimulated with touch or voice, and (c) look away when their gaze is engaged. Certainly such infants are hard to care for, putting bonding and attachment with a caregiver at risk.

The difficulty in establishing a clear pattern of effects is due, in part, to methodological difficulties, sample selection in the research, and the existence of confounding variables such as prenatal polydrug exposure (Lester et al., 1991). Before discussing the research results, it is helpful to have a basic understanding of the measures used.

Methodology

I undertook a comprehensive review of empirical studies of cocaine-exposed neonates' behavior to compare the neurobehavioral results (Sparks, 1990). To be included, studies had to have a comparison group of nonexposed infants, describe behaviors measured as neurobehavioral or behavioral, describe their method of observation, and present results of behavioral assessment. Only 9 of the original 88 studies identified by on-line database search and reference lists met these criteria. Of the studies that met the criteria (Anday et al., 1989; Ahmed, Spong, Geringer, Mou, & Maulik, 1989; Chasnoff, Burns, Schnoll, & Burns, 1985; Chasnoff, Burns, & Burns, 1987; Chasnoff, Griffith, MacGregor, Dirkes, & Burns, 1989; Chasnoff, Lewis, Griffith, & Wiley, 1989; Cherukuri, Minkoff, Feldman, Parekh, & Glass, 1988; Dixon, Coen, & Crutchfield, 1987; Fulroth et al., 1989), four behavioral measures were used: the Neonatal Behavioral Assessment Scale (NBAS) (Brazelton, 1984), Neonatal Abstinence Scoring System (Finnegan, 1985), observation, and electrophysiologic response. Because most studies of newborn behavior affected by prenatal drug exposure used the dissimilar measures of the NBAS and the Abstinence Scoring, these two instruments are described here in some detail to help the reader evaluate results.

The *Neonatal Behavioral Assessment Scale* (NBAS) (Brazelton, 1984), the most widely used behavioral assessment procedure for newborn infants, was originally devised for use with healthy full-term infants. The NBAS produces data on 28 standard behavioral items. Lester (1984) reduced the items into 7 clusters that represent constructs of neonatal behavior: (1) *habituation,* the ability to respond to and then inhibit responding to a discrete stimulus while asleep; (2) *orientation,* the quality of the alert states and the ability to attend to visual and auditory stimuli while alert; (3) *motor* performance and the quality of movement and tone; (4) *range of state,* a measure of the general arousal level or arousability of the infant; (5) *regulation of state,* how the infant responds when aroused; (6) *autonomic,* signs of stress related to homeostatic adjustments of the nervous system; and (7) *reflexes.* The infant's NBAS score is based on "best" performance, not average performance. The optimal time for testing is 3 days of age; it may be given only once or repeated to look for improvement, but there are no specified intervals for readministration of the test.

Griffith (1988) categorized cocaine-exposed infants into four behavioral categories while they were undergoing the 20-minute NBAS at the newborn period, at 1 week of age, and at 1 month of age: (1) those who never wake up; (2) those who never awaken but who show signs of distress throughout the exam; (3) those who vacillate between sleep states and cry states; and (4) those who sleep and cry but who have brief periods of alertness. By 1 month of age there is considerable improvement in the orientation abilities and state control abilities of the cocaine-exposed infants, but their performance is still significantly poorer than their drug-free counterparts. Griffith points out, however, that there is considerable variability from infant to infant with regard to both the severity of the initial response deficiencies and the rate of recovery.

The *Neonatal Abstinence Scoring System* (Finnegan, 1985) was developed to monitor the withdrawal symptoms of infants born to heroin- and methadone-dependent mothers for the purpose of pharmacotherapeutic intervention. Heroin and methadone are opiates and physical withdrawal symptoms are expected. The Abstinence Score lists 21 symptoms most commonly seen in the passively addicted neonate. Each withdrawal symptom and its associated degree of severity has been assigned a score. Infants are assessed 2 hours after birth and then every 4 hours. A score of eight or greater for three consecutive scorings is reason to consider pharmacotherapy for withdrawal symptoms. It is divided into three sections: *central nervous system disturbances, metabolic/vasomotor/respiratory disturbances,* and *gastrointestinal disturbances.* Infants prenatally exposed to cocaine, but not to heroin or methadone, do not have classic physical withdrawal symptoms and are seldom medicated at birth. (Medication interferes with an infant's important natural interactions at birth.) Neonatal Abstinence Scoring is not an appropriate test for children prenatally exposed to nonopiate drugs.

Measurement Problems

Several problems emerge from this review. First, the number of studies is small, and the results reported show little consistency. Second, differences in methodologies for measuring behavior contribute to the apparent lack of consistency. The purpose of abstinence scoring is to medicate appropriately infants who have withdrawal symptoms; all items are considered to be abnormal. On the other hand, the NBAS was standardized on normal infants. Items range on either side of normal from hypofunction to hyperfunction. Another important methodological difference concerns examiner bias; some of the assessors knew whether the infant was drug-exposed.

Based on the research reviewed and summarized in Table 3–2, it appears that cocaine-exposed neonates have behaviors in specific areas that may differentiate them from non-cocaine-exposed neonates. Behaviors most likely to differentiate the two groups are in the areas of orientation, involving visual and auditory response, and of motor development, involving muscle tone. Also consistent are behaviors in the areas of state control. How these behaviors of infancy translate into long-term behaviors that interfere with language and learning remains unclear.

Long-Term Behavioral Effects

Very little information regarding the long-term outcome of the cocaine-exposed infant is available because crack cocaine use has been prevalent only since approximately 1984, and some time elapsed before good studies were designed to measure exposed childrens' behavior. Again the problem of meaningful measures is apparent. It appears that prenatal drug exposure does have predictable adverse effects on developmental processes that extend beyond the infancy period in many children, at least into the toddler years. Those effects are summarized in Table 3–3.

Table 3–2
Neurobehavioral risks of prenatal cocaine exposure in infancy

Irritability

Hypertonicity

Hypotonicity

Hyperactivity

Tremulousness

Deficiencies in state organization

Deficiencies in interactive abilities

Seizures

Table 3-3
Long-term effects of prenatal
cocaine exposure

Reduced head circumference

Reduced self-regulation

Distractible

Less representational play

Flat affect

Attachment problems

Quantitative Measures

Chasnoff et al. (1992) used traditional methods of standardized test measurement. They have followed from birth a cohort of drug-exposed children whose mothers have sought recovery for themselves and intervention for their children. The mothers had prenatal care, good nutrition, and medical and developmental assessment and management which reduced greatly the number of risk factors beyond drug exposure; thus their study sample is a special group and not necessarily typical. Furthermore, their sample groups were exposed to polydrugs, that is, a group of infants exposed to cocaine and other drugs plus alcohol were compared to a group exposed to other drugs plus alcohol without cocaine. A control group had no drug exposure. The children have been assessed at 3, 6, 12, 18, and 24 months. Development was measured by both the Mental Developmental Index (MDI) and the Psychomotor Developmental Index (PDI) of the Bayley Scales of Infant Development (Bayley, 1969). Head circumference was correlated with cocaine exposure at 12, 18, and 24 months, but not below 12 months. There were relatively few significant differences among the three groups on either the MDI or the PDI at 2 years of age. The authors speculate, however, that the Bayley Scales may not provide an accurate assessment of the problems of some drug-exposed children. For example, drug-exposed infants are reported to have difficulties with self-regulation (Chasnoff, 1992b). If the assessor reduces stimulation and focuses the child's attention during the testing procedure, difficulty with self-regulation may not be apparent. Test situations may actually mask some of the self-regulatory difficulties experienced by cocaine- and other drug-exposed children. The authors speculate further that the manifestations of drug exposure may become evident later as these children must engage in increasingly complex thinking.

Observation

Another group of researchers (Howard, Beckwith, Rodning, & Kropenske, 1989; Rodning, Beckwith, & Howard, 1990) used observational methods in the belief that developmental and intelligence tests alone are inadequate in demonstrating the subtle deficits that would be most common in drug-exposed children. Developmental scores for their sample of drug-exposed children were consistent with those of Chasnoff et al. (1992); they agree that drug-exposed children can appear developmentally normal when externally structured and monitored by adults, as is the case with standardized tests. The capacities of children to meet daily challenges by actively engaging their environment, adapting their behaviors to the challenges in the environment, and initiating changes in the environment to meet their own needs are salient dimensions of behavior not captured in the scoring of standardized developmental tests. Rodning et al. (1990) compared drug-exposed 18-month-old toddlers to a sample of high-risk preterm toddlers. The setting was an unstructured free play situation that required self-organization, self-initiation, and follow-through without the assistance of the examiner to guide the task.

Actions that represent a simple functional occurrence are intentional actions that indicate the child's awareness of events in his or her environment. The salient function of play activity in the development of children underscores the importance of understanding what children are communicating through their actions and behaviors (Rodning et al., 1990). The drug-exposed children showed striking deficits in play. They had significantly less representational play than the high-risk preterm children. For the majority of drug-exposed children play was characterized by scattering, batting, and picking up and putting down the toys rather than sustained combining of toys, fantasy play, or curious exploration. Representational play events, such as combing hair, stirring a pot, and sitting a doll at a table, were significantly less frequent and less varied in the drug-exposed group than the comparison group (Howard et al., 1989).

The formation and organization of the toddler's attachment relationship with his or her caregivers and subsequently with others is another important issue in the social and emotional development of toddlers. The relationship that forms between the child and caregiver during the first year of life forms a pattern that influences the child's approach to intellectual, social, and emotional situations. As discussed in Chapter 2, when the pattern of organization is secure, the child can rely on the caregiver's presence for physical and psychological comfort. Arising out of this security, the child can explore the world, be goal directed, and persevere in mastering tasks, confident that the caregiver will be accessible when needed. When the pattern of organization is insecure, the child is not confident about the caregiver's availability or effectiveness in providing safety and protection. Thus, insecure children are preoccupied with monitoring the activity of their caregiver, and consequently are less free to explore and interact in the larger world. Howard et al. (1989) compared drug-exposed and preterm children using the Strange Situation paradigm (Ainsworth, Blehar, Waters, & Wall, 1978). This procedure places a mild stress on the child through a series of separations and reunions with the caregiver in an unfamiliar setting and with an unfamiliar adult present. The organization of the relationship between the child and caregiver is demonstrated in the reunions in the child's need for and effort to obtain proximity to the caregiver, to maintain close contact with the caregiver, or, on the other hand, to avoid interaction with the caregiver and to resist interaction when the child and caregiver are already in contact. Again the drug-exposed children had deviant behaviors. The drug-exposed children did not show the strong feelings of pleasure, anger, and distress in relation to novel toys and the caregiver's departure and return that the attachment assessment was designed to elicit. These children lacked clear affective cues, intentionality, and organized strategies toward their caregivers. Their affect was flat. Moreover, the majority of drug-exposed children had insecure attachments characterized by disorganization rather than organized patterns of avoidance or ambivalence. The theme of disorganization was present in each of the developmental areas assessed, cognitive, social, and affective.

The highest percentage of insecure drug-exposed toddlers was in the subgroup being raised by their biological mothers. In all but one case, these mothers continued to abuse drugs. The majority of drug-exposed toddlers reared by extended family members and foster mothers were secure, and this percentage of security was not significantly different from the percentage of security in the preterm comparison group. The primacy of satisfying the addiction over the welfare of themselves and their children, the impairment from chronic drug use, and the consequent unavailability of mothers on a high, or coming down from a high, suggest that the addicted mothers' ability to be psychologically responsive is greatly impaired despite their often best intentions to do otherwise (Rodning et al., 1990).

◼️ SUMMARY

Although the media portrays children who are drug-exposed as doomed, most exposed infants are unaffected. Affected infants exposed prenatally to cocaine appear most often to be irritable and stiff, but those symptoms appear to be transient and do not last into the toddler years. A more important diagnostic sign is reduced head circumference, because it designates brain size. Neurobehavioral effects in newborns are well documented, but the long-term effects of prenatal cocaine exposure are still unclear. An important inference for communication specialists is: Since a link between representational play and language acquisition has been demonstrated, we can also anticipate a risk for problems in language development for the drug-exposed children at later ages. Other inferences concerning treatment approaches will be explored in Chapter 4.

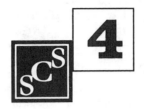

Interventions for Children Exposed to Cocaine

■ MARIO'S STORY

Mario, an African-American child, was seen by a multidisciplinary team when he was 26 months old. His mother, Monica, had used crack cocaine throughout her pregnancy with him and was seeking recovery. She requested the evaluation because she thinks that Mario is behind in his language and speech. Mario has a sister, age 9, and a baby brother, age 9 months, neither of whom were reported to be exposed to crack prenatally. The family is supported by public assistance; there has never been a father or adult male in the home. Housing has been especially difficult to find for this family. They live in a public housing complex where crack cocaine is sold and used openly. The following are excerpts from the oral reports given at the concluding diagnostic team meeting (Multiclinic, 1991).

Occupational Therapy

Mario lacked experience with many of the test items, such as scissors and beads. His eye-hand coordination seemed to be okay with instruction and repetition, but his fine motor skills were at about 17 months. During the feeding assessment he was noted to drool. He lacked lip closure and rotary chewing. He did not have a supinating elbow. He has several broken teeth. He does not like different textures and had a high degree of sensitivity around his mouth. Several reflexes that should have been integrated are not — such as the asymmetrical tonic neck reflex. He did not show normal labyrinthine or Landau responses. On the Peabody Developmental Motor Scale he was at the 20.4 month level. He responded to both nonverbal and verbal imitation. I would say that he has soft neurological signs (minimal symptoms of neurological disorder). I was impressed by the trust he showed with me. He wouldn't engage with pictures or anything I had to say about pictures.

Audiology

Mario has had an ear infection about every other month of his life and has had several courses of antibiotics. Right now he has flat tracings on tympanometry, which indicates fluid in the middle ear. On sound field testing he had thresholds at 35 dB when I tested him at 24 months. After a course of antibiotics, his thresholds went down to 15 dB at 26 months. He is certainly at risk for fluctuating hearing loss. The hearing loss he has experienced could have an impact on his difficulty with speech and language.

Speech-Language Pathology

Mario came to the speech room three times for his evaluation. The first time he played with the toys and warmed up to the situation. He was mostly mute but did speak two words. I watched him talk with his mom. She got close to him and at eye level and she used some expansions; when Mario said "ball," she said "throw the ball." Most of the time she was directive and commanding; when she was, Mario withdrew and reacted violently. Mario's speech is jargon-like. His intonation pattern is like speech but the words are unintelligible; his speech is somewhat like that of an 18-month-old child. On the Bayley Scale of Infant Development Mental Developmental Index his score was in the 17–19 month range. He could follow two short directions. His play showed short isolated pretend activities.

The second visit I put him in a preschool group, and his behavior did not change with the increased stimulation. He still made his wants known nonverbally, like holding up his cup for juice, frowning and pushing when children intruded on his toys. He would not let me look in his mouth; he seems to be hypersensitive there. He is very interested in food and his quickest reactions involved food.

Music Therapy

Mario seemed to understand cause and effect; he turned the omnichord button on and off to make it play. He played rhythmically and age-appropriately.

Home Visitor-Interventionist

Because Monica was on crack when Mario was born, I've been seeing her for our high-risk infant program. Touch has always been stressful for Mario. His mother has had a hard time with him for bathing, holding, diapering, and dressing him. She sees his speech and language problem as his only problem. My job has been to help her to identify his cues so she could respond to him and to learn how to hold him —to stimulate him without overstimulating him. I have also worked on helping her to deal with her feelings of guilt and rejection.

Substance Abuse Counselor

Before Monica went into recovery, the house was turned over to crack. After the crack times, the house was turned over to sleep. There was no time for nurturing children or for even the rudiments of cleanliness or housekeeping. There is a saying on the street that crack takes away "heart" — the part of you that cares about other people or anything else but crack. Monica voices deep guilt and remorse over this time. My job has been to help Monica with her recovery and staying sober. Her attitude has changed and her mothering skills have improved, although she feels tied down by her children.

Mother

(Response to question: What do you hope for your children?) I hope for a better life for them than we had — where they don't have to be on ADC (Aid to Dependent Children). So they don't have to be on drugs or live in a drug area.

(Question: How are things where you live?) Drugs are everywhere. Standing outside all drugged up. My daughter sees 'em sell it. In the summer I have to bring them in early. It's wild out there. It's very hard not to use it when that's all people do around you. 'Specially in an area when that's all there is and that's all people do. Can't just say no like that. Sometimes you can wake up in the morning and taste it. It's a fight not to use it. I'm fine when I'm busy. I know what I'm going to do and what I have to do. I have to find another place and a job — one thing at a time. A job then move. That's my first goal — that's what I'm thinking now. You get flustered when you think of all the things to do at once — when you know you have to do it and when that don't work like you want it to, it's kind of depressing.

(Question: What's the hardest thing about crack?) Staying off it. That's the hardest part.

Recommendations by the Diagnostic Team

1. Preschool experience for Mario either in a classroom for the speech and language impaired or in a classroom where he would have consultative services by the speech-language pathologist and the occupational therapist.

2. Continued counseling, education, and support for Monica.
3. Hearing monitoring and medical follow-up when appropriate.

Barriers to Recommendations

1. **Transportation.** It was unrealistic to recommend preschool for Mario when there was no transportation for him. No matter how good the program available for him, it was useless if he could not get there.
2. **Daycare.** There is no daycare available for Monica so that she can participate in any groups without her children with her — including drug counseling. Any service recommended for this family would have to go to the family as a home-based service. The home-visitor interventionist will have to conclude services when the baby is 1 year old — in 3 months — because of the program structure; Mario was already too old for the service.

It was also unlikely that Monica would be able to follow up with recommendations for Mario's hearing status, even though it was free, for the same reasons — no transportation or child care is available.

Outcome

Unfortunately, a year and a half later, Monica lost her fight to stay sober. She disappeared into the drug underground. Her children were taken in by relatives. Mario did not receive the early intervention recommended for him. He will go to school with a speech and language impairment.

■◻ BOBBY'S STORY

Bobby, also African-American, was born at 26 weeks gestation to a woman who had no prenatal care. He could hardly have had a rougher beginning. He weighed 900 grams. (Very low birth weight is 1500 grams and under.) He had a positive urine screen for cocaine at birth. Complications of his prematurity included a grade III intraventricular hemorrhage (bleeding into the fluid filled spaces of the brain which may cause severe brain damage resulting in cerebral palsy; grade IV is the highest designation), respiratory distress syndrome (a pulmonary disorder of premature infants caused by lack of surfactant in the lungs needed to keep the air sacs in the lungs open, which may lead to the chronic condition of bronchopulmonary dysplasia), and apnea of prematurity (prolonged pause in respiration often accompanied by a slowing of the heart rate) (Blackman, 1984). He was placed on a ventilator to breathe for him, and he remained on the ventilator for 4 weeks. Infants who are ventilated must be fed intravenously through a tube which is passed through the mouth or nose into the stomach (Schultz, 1984). His hospital stay was further complicated by a case of enterococcal bacteremia, a strep infection of the intestinal tract. His mother abandoned him at the hospital.

At 4 months of age, Bobby was discharged from the hospital in the foster care of a special care nursery nurse who had cared for him. She and her family of a husband and two older children are the only family Bobby has known; they formally adopted him at the age of 3. In addition to the stable and loving home environment they provided, Bobby received early and appropriate interventions, which are briefly described here (Lopacki, 1992, personal communication).

Hearing

Auditory brain response (ABR) testing done before Bobby left the hospital at 4 months revealed mildly abnormal tracings. ABR is a test of the integrity of the auditory mechanism, not hearing perception, and it does not require the cooperation of the infant, as does behavioral audiometry (Sparks, Clark, Erickson, & Oas, 1990). He had repeated bouts of otitis media and underwent a myringotomy with pressure equalization tubes placed in his ears at age 2. The procedure was repeated at age 3. At age 4 he began a course of prophylactic antibiotics for his ear infections. A test of hearing perception at age 4 revealed hearing within normal limits.

Physical Therapy

Bobby received physical therapy intermittently from the first year of his life for his hypertonic lower extremities and his hypotonic trunk.

Developmental Psychology

Bobby's mother sought and received advice about ways to calm him and ways to help him to focus his attention. She was helped to limit stimulation because he tended to be "extraordinarily active" about age 2. A limited attention span was also noted at that age.

Speech and Language Therapy

Bobby began speech and language therapy at age 2 because verbal language was nonexistent. He received individual traditional language therapy once per week until his expressive language emerged, at which time the sessions were cut to two times per month. At age 4 his language skills were within normal limits; only some articulation problems remain. He continues to see the speech-language pathologist approximately once per month for articulation therapy.

Preschool Education.

The speech-language pathologist suggested to Bobby's mother that he go to a specialized preschool where there were few children per teacher. The school experience proved to be an excellent one for Bobby. At age 4 he will go to a regular prekindergarten.

Outcome

Bobby appears to have caught up with his age peers at age 4 despite nearly overwhelming odds. He is called the "miracle baby" by his family and interventionists (Lopacki, 1992, personal communication). Certainly, he had advantages that other infants, notably Mario, do not have.

What Makes a Difference?

Why, then, is Bobby considered essentially normal at age 4 while Mario has deficits that may or may not be long lasting? What accounts for the difference in outcome for these two children? Two things were instrumental in helping Bobby to overcome his monumental physical problems at birth and catch up by age 4, and by the same token, these same factors contributed to Mario's decline in development: parenting and early intervention. In this chapter we will examine those factors and the interaction between them. The earliest intervention is intervention to help the caregiver with parenting. Later, when the child gets to school, specific techniques can aid attention and learning.

■ INFERENCES FROM RESEARCH

Some important research findings from the previous chapter will serve to structure our intervention strategies.

- Most children exposed to cocaine prenatally are unaffected.
- Early intervention, appropriate for other high-risk children, works for drug-exposed children.
- Neurobehavioral difficulties seen most often in drug-exposed children are that they are irritable and stiff as newborns. These patterns are transient and seldom last beyond infancy.
- Newborns show difficulties in self-regulation. Self-regulation problems may last into childhood.
- Drug-exposed infants catch up to nonexposed infants in birth weight and length.
- Drug-exposed infants have head circumferences that may be significantly smaller than nonexposed infants. Head circumference indicates brain size and is a predictor of mental ability.
- Psychomotor Developmental Index Scores on the Bayley Scales of Infant Development show no significant difference between exposed children and nonexposed children at 18 months of age.
- Mental Developmental Index Scores on the Bayley Scales of Infant Development show a decline for cocaine-exposed children at 18 months. However, nonexposed children from the same low socioeconomic environment also show a decline in scores at 18 months. The decline in scores is attributable to *language* items on the Bayley Scales.
- Children exposed to cocaine have more difficulty with verbal and nonverbal reasoning than nonexposed children.
- Evaluators rate children exposed to cocaine at ages 3 to 5 to have more distractability, increased activity level, and more difficulty with sound discrimination than nonexposed children. Exposed children also tend to prefer easy tasks and give up on tasks early. Articulation problems were also evident, but they were not significantly different from nonexposed children in the same environment.
- Mothers of the cocaine-exposed children rated their children's behavior as being socially withdrawn, being depressed, being aggressive, being destructive, and having sleep and somatic problems.
- Cocaine-exposed children are not necessarily retarded, nor do they show classic signs of learning disability.

■ Characteristics of children exposed to cocaine as they grow into childhood are low threshold for overstimulation, low threshold for frustration, withdrawal from stressful situations, and increasing rates of activity/impulsivity.

■ Children exposed to cocaine, especially if raised in a home where their caregivers are using drugs, tend to have problems of attachment and trust with their caregivers.

■ Caregiver's addiction has a negative impact on the caregiver-child relationship in a cycle; the poorer the care given the less confident the caregiver becomes in her ability to parent effectively.

Conceptual Framework

Three principles guide our intervention strategies for cocaine-exposed children, given the research to date:

1. Evaluate each child's threshold for controlling his or her self-regulation.
2. Work toward the child's understanding his or her own threshold and help the child to take steps to regulate himself or herself. Regulation must begin from the outside, from those in the environment, and then be internalized.
3. Work not only with the child but with the caregiver to build confidence, attachment, and trust in both members of the dyad.

For these principles to work, we must look to the structure of the learning environment, whether it is in the home with the caregiver, in special services, or in the classroom, and the individual child's interaction with that environment (setting and people). Some general guidelines specific to age groups follow.

■ INFANCY

Assessment

Normative infant tests can be used to ascertain eligibility for early intervention; all tests should be adjusted for age during the first year if the infant is premature. The test used most often for research with newborns exposed to drugs is the Neonatal Behavior Assessment Scales (NBAS)

(Brazelton, 1984). The test's organization was discussed in the previous chapter. The purpose of the NBAS is to assess organization in the full-term infant. For premature or small-for-gestational age infants, the Assessment of Preterm Infant Behavior (Als, Lester, Tronick, & Brazelton, 1982), or APIB, was developed. The infant's level of functioning is observed as well as his or her threshold for disorganization. The APIB is a comprehensive tool for evaluating the preterm infant's autonomic, motor, self-regulatory, attentional, and interactional abilities. It assesses behavioral capacities and organizational level from approximately 28 to 40 weeks of gestational age and is designed to answer the following questions (Sparks, 1989; VandenBurg, 1985):

- When, and with what help, does the infant function smoothly?
- How much and what kinds of stress and frustration are seen in the infant?
- How much energy does the infant have available for smooth functioning?
- How much handling can the infant tolerate before losing control?
- Is the infant's homeostatic balance easily disrupted?
- What strategies does the infant exhibit to avoid losing control?
- What support is necessary to help the infant to maintain self-control?

More recently, Als and her colleagues (Als, Duffy, & McAnulty, 1992) developed the Neonatal Individualized Developmental Care and Assessment Program (NIDCAP) and are training health care providers in its use. The approach is to observe the newborn for behavioral cues of stress and for cues of emerging capacities of self-regulation in order to structure care in such a way that stress is maximally diminished and self-regulatory capacity is maximally supported. This new means of observation should be invaluable in providing ways to structure the infant's environment based on the individual infant's cues.

Equal emphasis must be given to qualities of the caregiver and the quantity and quality of the interaction between the infant and caregiver. Caregiver observation instruments are listed in Appendix A (Sparks et al., 1990).

Intervention

Infants exposed to drugs may be very irritable to very passive, or they may have no problems with state control. Irritable infants can reach a frantic-cry state very quickly, which should be avoided by quick caregiver response and soothing. Swaddling should be used first. The caregiver should swaddle the infant with her arms in the midline position to counteract the "W" position of the arms that is typically seen in babies with poor muscle tone. Swaddling allows the infant to control excess motor activity so she can stay organized. If swaddling does not calm the infant, a pacifier may be offered, although the frantic-crying infant is frequently not organized enough to even suck on the pacifier. If those measures do not work, the infant can be held closely and rocked, especially in the vertical position. Caregivers should be shown how to monitor their interactions by being alert to signs of stress and giving the infant time out to recover control (see Tables 4–1 and 4–2). For example, when

TABLE 4–1

Signs of stress in newborn

Gaze aversion	Frowning or worried look
Yawning	Motor agitation
Sneezing	Grunting
Skin color change	Gagging
Hiccups	Spitting up
Furrowing brow	Irregular breathing
Irregular heart beat	

Source: From Lewis, K. D., Bennett, B., & Schmeder, N. H. (1989). The care of infants menaced by cocaine abuse. *Maternal Child Nursing, 14*(5), 324–329, reproduced with permission.

TABLE 4–2

Strategies to reduce stress and promote interaction

Stop activity that produces stress reaction. Give time-out.

Provide firm, strong touch.

Swaddle infant with arms close to body.

Pacifier.

Warm bath.

Vertical rocking.

Adjust stimuli in response to infant cues.

Source: From Lewis, K. D., Bennett, B., & Schmeder, N. H. (1989). The care of infants menaced by cocaine abuse. *Maternal Child Nursing, 14*(5), 324–329, reproduced with permission.

an infant averts her eyes from those of the caregiver, the caregiver may want to follow the infant's eyes and entice the infant to come back into the interaction. Caregivers of infants exposed to drugs should be shown how to allow the infant to recover and come back into the interaction in her own good time.

Interaction should take place during quiet alert, not hyperalert, states. The infant may require swaddling and a pacifier to reach a quiet responsive state. Caregivers should be shown how to introduce stimuli in one dimension at a time — voice only or face only, and then work up to voice and face and touch. The infant should guide the caregiver. Her cues will indicate what she can tolerate, likes, or dislikes. When the infant is calm, she can be unwrapped to allow her to become used to controlling her own body movement. Then she can be reswaddled if and when she begins to lose control again, for example, if she begins to show fussy, diffuse movements (Lewis, Bennett, & Schmeder, 1989).

Some infants exposed to drugs show gastrointestinal difficulties throughout their first year of life, which tend to increase irritability and discomfort. The infants may also sleep for long periods of time and thus be at risk for inadequate nutrition. They should be wakened for feedings. Table 4–3 shows some common oral-motor behaviors and interventions for facilitating feedings (Lewis et al., 1989).

Caregivers will be affected by infant irritability, which may result in frustration and feelings of inadequacy in the mothering role and infant-caregiver attachment. If the caregiver is made aware of what to expect in the infant's behavior, negative judgments about the infant can be reduced.

TABLE 4–3
Feeding behaviors and interventions

Behaviors	Interventions
Poor suck/swallow pattern	Hold infant in sitting position with arms forward, slight flexion.
Poor tongue stabilization in midline	
Tongue thrust	Keep chin tucked down.
Tongue tremors	Support chin and cheek with your hand.
	Play soft, rhythmic music.
	Allow resting during feeding.

Source: From Lewis, K. D., Bennett, B., & Schmeder, N. H. (1989). The care of infants menaced by cocaine abuse. *Maternal Child Nursing, 14*(5), 324–329, reproduced with permission.

▪️ TODDLERS AND SCHOOL-AGE CHILDREN

Assessment

Service providers and teachers may use any normative or critierion-referenced test appropriate for the child's age and the purpose for testing, for example, certifying eligibility for service or establishing intervention goals. As was pointed out in the previous chapter, normative tests do not give a true picture of behavior. Structured observations during play and in an interaction with the caregiver are necessary parts of the assessment.

Structured Observation

Caregiver-Infant Interaction and Caregiver

A number of observation instruments are available to guide the provider in assessing caregiver attributes. Typically, observations are recorded on a checklist while observing the caregiver in interaction with the infant or through direct caregiver interview (Sparks, 1989). Many providers have made videotaping the caregiver and child in a free-play interaction for careful viewing later a standard part of assessment. Suggested instruments for observation are listed in Appendix A at the end of this book.

Play Scales

Structured observation instruments for use while the child is in free play are also available. Interpersonal behaviors and language markers are recorded during play with specified materials (Sparks, 1989).

ABC Approach

VanBremen (1992) has described this technique of structured observation. It is not a new concept for speech-language pathologists who are well versed in observing behaviors in the context of antecedent and consequent events. A behavioral log is kept for the primary purpose of finding the behavioral threshold for the child, that is, when does the child lose control? For example, an ABC behavioral log for a negative behavior includes:

- **A** is the antecedent event. What is the situation? What occurred just prior to the behavior in question? Was the antecedent particularly stressful?
- **B** is the behavior. What is the behavior in verifiable and quantifiable terms? What purpose does it serve for the child in inferential terms? For example, if the child is running around the room, what is the duration of the behavior? What accompanies the behavior (verbalization, crying, motor behavior)? What could be the purpose of the behavior (loss of control, attention gaining)?
- **C** are the consequent events. Who reacts to the behavior in question? What do they do? Do the consequent events help the child to regulate herself? Maintain the behavior? Increase the behavior?

The log can be kept in any form. It enhances observation by the caregiver, teacher, or service provider to focus on events that surround the behavior instead of just focusing on the behavior. A positive or controlled behavior may be reinforced by "catching" the child in the behavior and using positive reinforcement techniques of praise, that is, "You really stuck with that activity until you were finished. You should be proud of that."

Intervention

The following general guidelines are directed to the teacher or service provider who works with drug-exposed children individually or in groups. They come from two centers: (1) the National Association for Perinatal Addiction Research and Education (NAPARE) in downtown Chicago which has been following a group of over 200 infants who were born prenatally exposed to cocaine as well as to marijuana and alcohol (the program is described later in this chapter as a community-based program); and (2) the Los Angeles Unified School District's Prenatally Exposed to Drugs (PED) Program for 3- and 4-year-old children (Today's Challenge, 1989).

Use the Individual Family Service Plan (IFSP) Format

The best planning comes from a team that includes the caregiver, so that the child is treated consistently at home and at school. Identify the family concerns and assess the family needs, keeping in mind what has been discussed about the drug-using family in this book. The team should discuss all member's observations of the child's behavior and progress. Intervention is best achieved when all professionals concerned with the child and family are coordinated. To accomplish this successfully, time must be allotted for teachers to meet and plan with assistants and for support services to come together in a transdisciplinary model.

Plan Intervention Based on Observation

Planning is based on observation, whether ABC or some other structured observation is used. Plan a number of activities; you may need lots of trial and error to find activities that help a particular child to stay below his or her threshold of control. The manner in which a child uses language, social-emotional, cognitive, and motor skills during play, at transition time, and while engaged in self-help activities is important. Close observation of a child's behavior at these times permits understanding of how the child experiences stress, relieves tension, copes with obstacles, and reacts to change. It provides valuable information on how the child uses peers and adults to meet needs and solve problems.

Organize the Environment

Caregivers, teachers, and service providers must evaluate the child's environment for materials and events that enhance the child's capacity for control and self-regulation. A child's ability to predict and anticipate the order of daily activities reduces anxiety. Look at materials in the classroom and the structure of the day with the question of overstimulation in mind. Control the stimuli in a therapy situation to allow for maximum self-regulation. A setting in which classroom materials and equipment can be removed to reduce stimuli or added to enrich the activity is best. For older children, help them arrange materials in their desks or lockers, instead of leaving it to chance. Give them guidance about what goes where and label the compartments. Help caregivers to add as much structure to the home as possible.

The following are samples of ways to design the physical environment for the child prenatally exposed to drugs (*Strategies for Teaching Young Children Prenatally Exposed to Drugs*, 1990).

- ◼️ The room should be divided into several distinct areas or interest centers with well defined boundaries consisting of low shelves, screens, furniture, and so forth.

- Spaces within the class can also be clearly defined; the way furniture is used (four chairs and a table) or two places at an easel can indicate work areas for children. You can also use masking tape or contact paper over construction paper to section off tables, placemats, or carpet to define working spaces. Hula hoops can become movable boundaries for a child's individual activity.
- Area signs help children associate specific behaviors, activities, and materials with a particular space. Area signs are realistic drawings of materials or activities that can represent an area (a crayon for the art area). Pictures can be hung as mobiles from the ceiling or mounted on folders to stand up on a table.
- Material labels are objects, small pictures, and names of classroom items that can be used to key the items to areas where they are kept or used. Labeling shelves and places for use solves many classroom clean-up problems.
- "Child signs" are cards on which you put each child's name and picture (or symbol). They are used to designate personal spaces and belongings within the classroom.
- Traffic patterns should be well defined.
- Use materials on a rotating basis; do not have everything out at once. Displays of children's work should be changed routinely to reflect current activities.
- Open shelves can be covered with curtains, particularly if the teacher uses the area as a backdrop for teaching or group activities.
- Cuing techniques help children learn to use the environment in an orderly manner, such as procedure cards, footprints to designate numbers of children at a center or how to line-up, directional arrows for traffic patterns, or traffic lights to represent open or closed areas of the classroom (such as the bathroom).

Focus Attention

Children who have not attained control or self-regulation need to have individual help with focusing attention. Address the child by name and get eye contact or touch the child before giving a verbal command. You may need to help the child to read the teacher's cues by explaining what the teacher's look, body language, or gestures mean. Work from maximum assistance in focusing attention on a task, staying with the child until the task is completed to the best of his ability, to allowing some time for longer and longer periods of independent work. When a child seems to get out of control, remove him from the situaion and help him calm himself, get eye contact, sit next to him and make body contact, and give verbal reassurance.

Aid Decision Making

Provide daily opportunities to make small decisions and limited choices in play or other activities. To aid decision making, talk the child through to the consequences of his action. Work below the child's threshold of control and ask for small decisions, working up to large decisions, for example, from which color to use to choosing clothing to be worn outside. Use physical, concrete, and verbal cues to direct or redirect a child in an activity.

Make Daily Routines Predictable

Help caregivers to organize the child's day in some routine or predictable fashion. This is nearly impossible in a home where routines are built around obtaining drugs, using the drugs, and recovering from using drugs. The mother in recovery can also benefit from daily routines. Certainly the classroom routine and therapies can be structured in a predictable pattern. Reduce classroom interruptions as much as possible. Not all service providers need to come into the classroom weekly to interact with the children. These adults should develop a routine for reintroducing themselves and telling the children when they will appear again.

Structure Transitions

Managing transitions from activity to activity is particularly difficult for children prenatally exposed to drugs (VanBreman, 1992). Establish classroom routines with a minimum number of transitions. Give warning when a transition is coming, for example, "In 5 minutes we will put away the books and have our snack." Signals, such as a bell, can be used in the classroom. Special preparation is given to transition time, recognizing that it is one of the best times of the day to teach the child how to prepare for and cope with change.

Encourage Attachment

School should be a place where children exposed to drugs can form attachments with adults and learn to trust. It is particularly important for teachers and service providers to be there consistently and to keep turn-over to a minimum. In the early years, providing attachment is more important than any readiness or academic activities. These children need a teacher who realizes that a child becomes sensitive and aware of the needs and feelings of others only by repeatedly having his or her own needs met. The children should be encouraged to sit on a teacher's lap.

Keep Groups and Classes Small

The guidelines outlined here cannot be achieved in large classrooms or therapy groups. Children exposed to drugs focus best when they receive individual attention. Teacher to student ratios are ideally no larger than 1:4.

Co-Teach to Avoid Isolation and Burnout

Be careful of isolation when working with children exposed to drugs. Two teachers, a teacher and an aide, or one teacher and one provider, can do a better job of the ABC technique than can one alone. School providers and teachers working in a collaborative model can be invaluable to each other in observations to enhance their planning and intervention.

Use Whole Language Approaches

It is beyond the scope of this book to give a comprehensive view of the whole language approach to intervention. The reader is referred to Norris and Hoffman (in press). However, a useful strategy embedded in a whole language approach is children's story-telling. Encouraging children's stories not only facilitates language learning, but also allows children to unburden themselves about the things in their environment that concern them: fears, isolation, losses, and family relationships. It is not unusual to uncover abusive situations in childrens' stories. They must be dealt with, as with any suspicion of abuse, and reported to your supervisor or protective services.

Structure Communication Activities

All children learn language best through social interaction with significant individuals and through active exploration of their environment.

Drug-exposed children may be unable to verbalize their needs, wants, and fears and instead tend to express them through behavior such as banging, stomping, and shouting. They may also observe passively rather than verbally engage with other children in play. Use eye contact and give simple one-step directions, and gradually increase the number of steps in a direction. Provide the names of people, pets, food items, body parts, objects, feelings, and events in the process of conversation. Immediately respond to beginning attempts at verbal communication. Provide strategies to the child to appropriately express what she or he needs and wants.

Structure Play Activities

Play is the area where a child integrates learning communication, social-emotional, and motor skills. Through play, a child can learn to understand herself and her relation to others and the world around her. As a child grows and matures, her play involves increased communication skills, attention, concentration, and concept development. Give each child toys and areas in the classroom that are his or hers alone and do not have to be shared. It is important to provide models of play behavior if a child has not had them at home or with other children. Before play begins, model the toy choices with correct verbal cues. Follow the child's lead in play. Model interactive play and then provide opportunities for the child to play interactively in a safe environment with the adult available for assistance and reassurance. It may be necessary to model the pretend or dramatic play that is so important to preschoolers to sort out what is real and what is make-believe. Although it is often the best strategy to allow children to solve their own conflicts, for these children it is advisable to give some extra support to the child who lacks the developmental skills necessary to solve conflicts.

◼️ COMMUNITY-BASED COMPREHENSIVE PROGRAMS

The most highly recommended intervention model for children exposed to cocaine or other drugs who are living with the biologic mother is believed to be a comprehensive model program: The mother receives treatment for her addiction, and the child receives early intervention under the same administrative structure. There are many advantages to this model, one of which is that the overall goals are family goals;

the staffs of the programs have an opportunity for interaction to facilitate individual goals of the child and parent to enhance their interaction.

The following services should be included in a model program (Kumpfer, 1991):

- Staff that is trained and sensitive to pregnant addicts' issues.
- Provision of adequate physical, interpersonal, and social supports.
- Family involvement in therapy and child care.
- Obstetric, pediatric, and medical care for women and infants.
- Educational and vocational assistance.

A number of programs throughout the country are attempting this comprehensive approach. Unfortunately, most do not have sufficient funding for rigorous evaluation of their effectiveness (Kumpfer, 1991). Therefore, we must rely on the subjective evaluation of those involved, primarily from professional staff. Not every program can afford the comprehensive services outlined above, but many arrange to provide some combinations of services to mothers and their children.

One model program is the National Association for Perinatal Addiction Research and Education (NAPARE) program in Chicago, Illinois (Chasnoff, 1992b). Women who enter the program are addicted to cocaine and other drugs during pregnancy. They receive comprehensive prenatal and medical care and addiction treatment to reduce or eliminate their drug usage. After the birth, the women return with their children for early intervention and continued addiction treatment. The women who seek out such a program are obviously motivated to do something for themselves and for their children.

A weekly staffing is held for one child each week with the mother's drug counselor as part of the team. Even so, in this program as in others in which programs and goals are combined, the mother's treatment program and the child's early intervention program may have conflicts, especially over the mother's time commitment. For example, the early intervention staff want to have the mother attend school with her child, while the addiction treatment program considers attendance at their program to be a top priority. Such timing questions can be negotiated in staff meetings.

Goals for Intervention with the Caregiver in a Comprehensive Program

The primary goal of intervention with the mother is to improve her feelings of competence as a parent, that is, to give her experiences in which she is successful in parenting. According to VanBremen (1992), that means we must treat her as if she has the competence we want her to have. To do so, we must balance our goals for her as a parent with her goals in recovery treatment. We must be careful to evaluate her status in the recovery process; she may have to look inward for some time before she is ready to think of herself as a parent. All programs for parents must be aware of cultural differences and work within the culture of the parent, not the culture of the teacher or provider.

Guidelines for Intervention with the Caregiver in a Comprehensive Program

Some general guidelines for building competence with a recovering mother follow.

◼ Begin goal setting with the concerns of the mother. Ask her to think about what she is doing as a mother and what she sees as problems.

◼ Work toward togetherness in the classroom or therapy. The amount of time the mother spends with her child will be dictated in large part by her recovery program, but negotiate as much as you can. Attachment and interaction can only occur when the mother and child are together.

◼ Observe her with her child and find some competence. Even mothers most in need of help in parenting will have some behavior that can be pointed to as exemplary. Point it out to others.

◼ Have play groups with mothers and their children (Klein & Briggs, 1987). Instead of using providers as models of behaviors, point out the positive behaviors of the mothers. You may attribute intention on the part of the mother when, perhaps, none exists. For example, a mother moves from in back of her child to face her in order to be more comfortable; the provider points out how that movement allowed a face-to-face position ("Notice how Angela moved so that Susan can see her face and how happy Susan looks now").

◼ Use videotape of group and individual sessions with the children. As you watch the videotape with the mother, point out all her positive behaviors. Klein, Briggs, and Huffman (1988) discuss videotape strategies for use in individual and group sessions with low-socioeconomic-status mothers and their infants.

Their goals are to convey information and to enhance and encourage caregivers' use of positive communicative interactions with their infants by replaying segments over and over to point out positive interactions between mother and child.

■ Have the mothers make toys for the children. Being able to complete a task that will benefit their children is a successful technique to build confidence.

■ Provide model strategies for play with children. Mothers may not have a repertoire of play strategies stemming from the way they were parented. If possible, the play strategies should come from another mother, but reciting nursery rhymes and finger plays, and reading books, can be initiated by the provider or teacher.

■ Help the mother to achieve literacy. Twelve-step recovery programs require reading and writing, and the programs assume literacy. Whatever you can do to begin or enhance the mother's literacy will boost her self-confidence as a parent and as a person.

■❏ SUMMARY

At the beginning of this chapter we discussed two cocaine-exposed children and asked what accounted for the difference in their outcomes at 4 years of age. The child with devastating physical problems at birth overcame them to start school as an essentially normal child; the other child seemed to fall farther and farther behind in development. Our research base is scanty, but it is adequate for two important principles to emerge: We can make a difference with drug-exposed children by helping their parents to parent effectively and by providing appropriate early intervention.

5

Fetal Alcohol Syndrome and Fetal Alcohol Effects

Alcohol-related congenital disorders are now recognized as the leading known cause of mental retardation in the United States (Abel & Sokol, 1987). The anomalies related to maternal drinking during pregnancy range from a severe recognizable pattern called fetal alcohol syndrome (FAS) to a condition in which not all the physical or behavioral symptoms of FAS are displayed, called fetal alcohol effect (FAE). There is some controversy concerning whether there are two disorders, FAS and FAE, or whether FAS and FAE are actually the extremes of a contiuum of a single condition: alcohol-related disorder. If a distinction need not be made between FAS and FAE, the term alcohol-related disorder will be used here to include both FAS and FAE.

A team of researchers has presented conclusive evidence (Streissguth, Aase, Clarren, Randels, LaDue, & Smith, 1991) that FAS is not just a childhood disorder; there is a predictable long-term progression of the disorder into adulthood in which maladaptive behaviors present the greatest challenge to management. Those maladaptive behaviors include predictable language disorders.

In this chapter, some common questions will be addressed: What are FAS and FAE? How common are they? Why do children have these conditions? How do I know if a child or adolescent in my school is affected by these disorders? Does it really matter if the diagnosis is alcohol-related? How can I get a diagnosis? What is my role in assessment? What can I expect of these children's language and speech? What happens as they get older? To gain a comprehensive understanding of the disorders, some background information on the action of alcohol is also provided.

◼ HISTORICAL PERSPECTIVE

Although alcohol has been suspected of causing congenital anomalies since Biblical times, "Behold thou shalt conceive and bear a son: now drink no wine or strong drink" (Judges 13:7), little research was done in modern times. Alcohol researchers were preoccupied with investigating the hypothesis of genetic damage in alcoholism, and the questionable status of offspring of alcoholics was often attributed to their chaotic home environment. In fact, some medical textbooks in the 1950s and 1960s claimed there were no harmful effects resulting from maternal alcohol use. Physicians were known to prescribe a drink before retiring for their pregnant patients for its calming effect.

Dorris (1989) chronicled the sparse knowledge of alcohol-related birth anomalies when his son Adam was born in 1968. That year, four French scientists published a modest research paper noting certain recurrent birth defects in 127 children of alcoholic parents. In 1974, the full fetal alcohol syndrome was described by Jones, Smith, Streissguth, and Myrianthopoulos. The meager research reports in the early years quickly gained momentum. By 1979, more than 200 FAS-related articles had been published. It was not until 1981 that the Surgeon General recommended that women who are pregnant or are considering pregnancy abstain from alcoholic beverages. By 1985, FAS-related professional documentation had increased to almost 2,000 articles, and it has grown exponentially since then.

◼ FETAL ALCOHOL SYNDROME

The three diagnostic criteria for the severe end of the contiuum of alcohol-related disorders that is FAS are growth deficiency, dysmorphology, and neurobehavioral effects. But prenatal alcohol exposure is not the only cause of the anomalies, so the diagnosis of FAS must also include information about prenatal alcohol exposure (Streissguth et al., 1991; Streissguth & LaDue, 1987; Streissguth, LaDue, & Randels, 1988). Diagnosis of FAS is a clinical judgment. There are no laboratory tests. For a diagnosis of FAS, there must be some manifestations in each of the three categories.

Growth Deficiency

Infants and Children

The growth deficiency is manifested in height, weight, and head circumference at birth, and catch-up growth is not seen in childhood. Children with FAS are usually below the third percentile for these growth parameters.

Adolescents and Adults

Height is the most severely affected growth parameter in adolescents and adults with FAS. For weight, a different pattern is manifest; relative to height, there is less growth deficiency for weight with increasing age, particularly after puberty. Girls may even become overweight and appear to be stocky. As children get older, microcephaly remains a prominent growth deficiency.

Dysmorphology

Infants and Children

Dysmorphology is impaired or abnormal structure. The characteristic face of FAS (Figure 5–1) includes several dysmorphic features. The eyes may have a prominent fold of skin in the inner corner, called epicanthal folds, and the eyes may be notably short from the inner to outer corners (palpebral fissures). The midface may be flat with a smooth and/or long philtrum, small chin, and thin upper lip. Not all of these features need appear at once. Other frequently seen dysmorphic features are prominent lateral palatal ridges, posterior rotation of the ears, and sensorineural hearing loss, in addition to otitis media (Church & Gerkin, 1988). The newborn profile includes a short, upturned nose, a convex philtral area, and a small receding chin. Features that appear occasionally are poorly formed ears, cleft lip or cleft palate, small teeth with faulty enamel, and

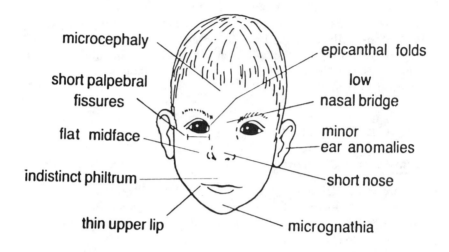

Figure 5-1
Features on the left are those most frequently seen in children with FAS. Those on the right are also seen with increased frequency in the normal population. From Little, R. E., & Streissguth, A. P. (1982). Alcohol: Pregnancy and the fetal alcohol syndrome. In *Alcohol use and its medical consequences: A comprehensive teaching program for biomedical education* (Unit 5). Project Cork of Dartmouth Medical School. (A slide teaching unit available from Milner-Fenwick, Inc., 2125 Greenspring Drive, Timonium, MD 21093.) Reproduced with permission.

limited joint movements. Other organ systems that may be affected are cardiac, renogenital, cutaneous, skeletal, and muscular (Clarren & Smith, 1978).

Adolescents and Adults

The facial features gradually become less distinctive with increasing age. Features sometimes take on a coarse appearance; the nose and chin grow and become more prominent. Abnormalities of the philtrum and lip remain useful diagnostic features in adolescents and adults. Other prominent facial characteristics are dental anomalies, including malformed teeth, malocclusions, poorly aligned teeth, and high arched palate. Skeletal anomalies are also quite prevalent, particularly finger anomalies, scoliosis, and short neck. Skeletal anomalies and postural problems should not be overlooked as diagnostic signs in older individuals.

Neurobehavioral Effects

Infants and Children

The neurobehavioral effects of prenatal alcohol, a manifestation of central nervous system damage, are produced at lower exposure levels than the dysmorphic or growth effects (Riley & Vorhees, 1986). These effects include tremulousness, delayed development, hyperactivity, attention deficits, memory problems, learning disabilities, intellectual deficits, and seizures (Clarren & Smith, 1978). Early IQ scores remain generally stable, although some children have been observed to raise their IQ scores considerably; the increased scores may be due to lack of reliability of test scores in very young children. Streissguth, Sampson, and Barr (1989a) studied children across a 10-year period and noted that the long-term effects, as measured by low IQ, are predictable for the most part from preschool IQ tests. However, IQ can be misleading as a predictor of adaptive functioning. Alcohol exposure has the strongest effect on processes such as reaction time, latency to respond, attention, and speed, suggesting some impairment in the central processing of information.

Adolescents and Adults

Intellectual impairment is observed into maturity. Adolescents and adults with alcohol-related disorders are consistently noted to function several years below their chronological age. No general tendency toward catching up is noted as individuals get older. In the early grades, the achievement test scores of these children are often at or near grade level, despite a lower IQ score. However, as the children grow older, the achievement scores peak and become more consistent with IQ scores. It should be noted that there are often score differences between ethnic and racial groups of FAS adolescents on standardized IQ and achievement tests (Streissguth et al., 1988).

■ FETAL ALCOHOL EFFECTS

FAE is much harder to recognize. The diagnostic criteria include prenatal alcohol exposure but not all of the physical or behavioral symptoms of FAS. The cognitive and behavioral characteristics of FAS and FAE are similar. Studies suggest a relationship between severity of physical characteristics and severity of mental retardation; thus children with a diagnosis of the full FAS would be expected to function more poorly, in general, than those with possible FAE (Streissguth, Landesman-Dwyer,

Martin, & Smith, 1980). However, there is considerable overlap between the IQ distributions of the two groups. Therefore, FAE can have equally serious implications for education (Burgess & Streissguth, 1990). One or two of the following constitute possible FAE.

1. Only growth deficiency.
2. Only a pattern of dysmorphology.
3. Only neurobehavioral effects.

"Possible FAE" is the term usually used for children who have some, but not enough of the characteristics to warrant diagnosis of FAS. For example, a child might be called FAE if she or he had growth deficiency and neurobehavioral characteristics but not facial dysmorphology. As Streissguth (1990) notes, the word "possible" refers only to etiology. The children's problems are real, not just possible.

■☐ INCIDENCE

A major misconception is that crack cocaine is the primary drug of abuse by pregnant women and is the drug that is most harmful to the newborn. In fact, estimates based on a recent national survey suggest that women were 16 times more likely to have used alcohol as cocaine during the pregnancy (National Institute on Drug Abuse, 1991); and alcohol, unlike cocaine, has proven harmful effects (Rinkel, 1992). The incidence of FAS is generally reported as 1 to 6 per 1,000 live births in the United States, but in their epidemiologic review, Little and Wendt (1991) reported a birth incidence in the United States and Canada that varies from 6 per 1,000 in an urban area to 121 per 1,000 in an isolated Native American community. The incidence of FAE is unknown but is probably two to three times as high as FAS. Alcohol-related birth anomalies can occur in every segment of society, as can alcoholism, and alcohol exposure should never be overlooked as a possibility because of the mother's race or class. The tendency of physicians who treat middle and upper class women to underreport cases of alcohol-related disorders is known as NIMO (not in my office). However, it is becoming increasingly evident that the expression of fetal alcohol effects is influenced by racial/ethnic origin and by socioeconomic status (SES). According to Little and Wendt (1991):

> American Indians have the highest rate of FAS in the Birth Defects Monitoring Program supported by the Centers for Disease Control (Chavez, Cordero, & Becerra, 1989). The rate for FAS in newborn black infants is also more than six times greater than for white infants. These discrepant

rates may reflect differential patterns of diagnosis or inherent susceptibility; the true reasons for the excess of cases are unknown. However, there is increasingly clear evidence of an interaction of SES with the relationship between maternal drinking and fetal effect. Poor women appear to have a higher risk of fetal alcohol effects than middle-class women (Streissguth & LaDue, 1985). Since the race and SES of subjects vary widely across the major longitudinal studies of drinking and pregnancy, it is not surprising that their results do not always agree. (p. 193)

The incidence of alcohol-related birth defects is related to the incidence of alcohol consumption in particular populations. The proportion of heavy drinkers in a society will increase as the mean alcohol consumption rate increases and decrease as it decreases. In societies that have a low mean consumption, a small percentage of the population will drink beyond a certain high level of consumption, but in a society where the mean consumption is high, the percentage of the population above that level will also be high (McKim, 1991). One implication of this relationship is that a society that has a high proportion of heavy drinkers will also have a high proportion of alcohol-related birth defects.

Risk

Risk is the potential to develop a disorder based on specific biological, environmental, or behavioral factors. Risk has been calculated for a population in Cleveland as 2.5% for FAS and 50% for FAE in pregnancies associated with heavy drinking (Sokol, Miller, & Reed, 1980). Risk can be increased or decreased by the concurrent use of other substances with alcohol; in fact, the effects of smoking appear to have an additive effect with heavy drinking (Little, 1977; Sokol et al., 1980), contributing to a nearly fourfold increase in risk of intrauterine growth retardation. On the other hand, there is evidence that substantially reducing alcohol or abstaining from alcohol during the last stages of pregnancy decreases the risk of adverse effect. The fetal risks involved in moderate or minimal alcohol consumption have not been established through research to date, nor has a safe level of maternal alcohol consumption.

CONCEPTUAL FRAMEWORK

Environmental vs. Genetic Causation

In the lexicon of congenital disorders, an important distinction is made between genotype and phenotype. *Genotype* refers to the actual genetic makeup of an individual: the DNA found in the genes that are contained on the chromosomes. *Phenotype* is the observable physiological and behavioral characteristics of an individual. We do not know by observing phenotypic features whether they are the result of the genotype or whether they are the result of an insult to the fetus that occurred during gestation. For example, cleft palate is a phenotypic feature with causes that include an aberrant gene (a genotypic cause) or an infectious agent such as rubella (an environmental cause).

FAS and FAE, like disorders attributable to other drugs taken by the mother during pregnancy, have an environmental rather than a genetic etiology. That is, the insult to the fetus occurs in the uterine environment during gestation after the genotype has been established at conception. Therefore, individuals with FAS or FAE cannot pass on any traits of the disorders to their children through their genes. The genotype is not affected by prenatal alcohol exposure, but the phenotype is affected during prenatal development. Etiology is clearly attributed to alcohol intake by the mother during pregnancy.

Paternal Relationship

The role of paternal drinking is less clear. Some prospective epidemiological studies have suggested that low birth weight is correlated with paternal alcohol consumption. Literature reviews by Little and Wendt (1991) and Phillips, Henderson, and Schenker (1989) concluded that there is no biological mechanism whereby the father's drinking could be responsible for the pattern of anomalies observed. There is no clear evidence of a mutagenic effect or of chromosomal damage. However, there is a growing animal literature which indicates that this question should not be ignored.

Alcohol as a Teratogen

A *teratogen* is a substance capable of producing death, malformations, growth deficiency, or behavioral aberrations as a result of prenatal exposure (Wilson, 1977). A behavioral teratogen is a substance that produces behavioral deviations as a result of prenatal exposure (Vorhees & Butcher, 1982). Perhaps the best known teratogen is thalidomide which was found to cause major limb malformations in children whose mothers took it during early pregnancy. During a short period in the early 1960s, 20% of the mothers who received the drug during the critical exposure period of pregnancy (McBride, 1977) produced babies with a degree of limb aberration, usually congenital absence of the limb. However, no known teratogen, including alcohol, has been shown to have a definite cause-and-effect connection with a specific type of abnormality; that is, the abnormality does not always appear when the teratogen is present, and when it does appear, its features are variable.

One reason that alcohol has been identified only recently as a teratogen is that not every woman who drinks heavily during pregnancy produces an affected child, and a woman who drinks very little may have an affected child. As Beck (1984) noted, society is of two minds about the risk of teratogens:

> If alcohol were any other powerful teratogen, it would have been banned as soon as it was linked with birth defects — as thalidomide was. Even if it were merely suspected of causing birth defects in concentrations as small as one part per billion — as dioxin is — the government would feel obliged to spend millions of dollars to protect people from contact with it. Even if it only damaged second-generation rats whose mothers were overdosed almost to death — as saccharin did — the government would require warnings to be posted.
>
> But because it's liquor that's killing the brain cells of unborn babies and distorting their growth, what we do is just hope that women who are pregnant or about to become pregnant will somehow get the message and act on it themselves. (p. 94)

(See Chapter 7 for prevention methods.)

Three factors must be considered in risks of teratogenicity:

◼️ *Time of Exposure.* Organ systems have different critical periods of development when cell division is most rapid and they are most vulnerable to teratogens. The brain has a relatively long critical period characterized by a complex series of specific critical periods for its different sections. Malformations probably are produced by high concentrations of alcohol at specific periods during the first trimester, when embryonic development of the central nervous system is taking place. Growth may be most vulnerable to heavy drinking during the second and third trimesters. Behavior disturbance and intellectual impairment may occur throughout pregnancy by chemical and structural disruption of the central nervous system in the first trimester, and in the second and third trimesters during the later period of cell divison associated with rapid brain growth and functional organization (Rosett, 1979).

◼️ *Dosage.* The neurobehavioral effects of prenatal alcohol exposure show, in general, a dose-response relationship; high levels of exposure are associated with large effects, whereas moderate levels of exposure are associated with more subtle effects. It is not clear whether the damage results from brief, high concentrations of alcohol at particular stages of development or whether FAS symptoms are caused by continuous consumption at low doses (McKim, 1991). (For an in-depth discussion of dose-related symptomatology, see Little and Wendt, 1991.) Some of the strongest predictors of later neurobehavioral deficits are binge drinking (five drinks or more on an occasion in the designated time period) and drinking in the period prior to pregnancy recognition (Streissguth, Sampson, & Barr, 1989).

Even moderate drinking has been shown to be associated with neurobehavior, notably IQ. Streissguth, Sampson, Barr, Darby, and Martin (1989) examined IQ at age 4 in relation to drinking and smoking in pregnancy in a large cohort study. Smoking was significantly related to low birth weight, but low birth weight did not predict IQ at age 4. However, prenatal alcohol exposure was significantly related to child IQ at age 4 in a relatively healthy, generally middle-class sample. Self-reported consumption of over three drinks a day on the average was associated with an average IQ decrement of almost five IQ points, after adjustment for a wide variety of other factors that also predict child IQ. This decrement represents an estimated tripling of the risk of subnormal intelligence for a child of "average background." For those 4-year-olds, the performance rather than verbal aspects of intelligence were most strongly correlated with prenatal alcohol exposure. The authors caution against using three drinks a day as a "threshold" for safety.

■ *Genotype of the Fetus and Genotype of the Mother.* Discrepancies in the studies of dosage may be attributable, in part, to differences in individual susceptibility. The mother's ability to detoxify alcohol is a possible factor in determining teratogenicity to her fetus, as is the susceptibility of an individual fetus to the teratogen.

So far, little is known about the interaction of the above factors in the expression of alcohol-related disorders. As we shall see in Chapter 9, the interactions of these variables make research extremely difficult.

■ ALCOHOL

Alcohol is a chemical term that covers a class of substances. *Ethanol* (ethyl alcohol) is what we drink. In the adult drinker, alcohol is absorbed in the digestive tract; it readily dissolves in water, and it may pass into the blood from the stomach and intestines, but it is absorbed most rapidly from the small intestine. Consequently, the peak blood level and the duration of action are determined by the speed with which alcohol gets through the stomach to the intestine. Alcohol is then distributed rather evenly throughout body water and crosses the blood-brain barrier as well as the placental barrier without difficulty. Consequently, alcohol levels in most tissues of the body, including the brain and the fetus, accurately reflect the blood alcohol level (BAL) of the drinker. BAL is a fraction denoting milligrams of alcohol per 100 milliliters of blood. It is possible to express this figure as a percentage by weight. For example, the BAL at which you are legally intoxicated in many jurisdictions is 80 mg alcohol in 100 ml of blood; that is 80 mg alcohol in 100,000 mg of blood, expressed as 0.08%.

Alcohol is metabolized mostly by the liver in two steps. First, alcohol is converted to acetaldehyde by the enzyme alcohol dehydrogenase. In the next step, acetaldehyde is converted into acetyl-coenzyme A, which is converted mainly into water and carbon dioxide through a process during which usable energy is released into the body. Alcohol metabolism can alter a great deal of body chemistry (McKim, 1991).

Effects on the User

Alcohol is classified as a sedative hypnotic drug. Like barbiturates and benzodiazepines, it reduces anxiety and inhibition and can produce behavioral sedation and coma with sufficient doses. At low doses it may produce a stimulant effect, and at higher doses it depresses the central nervous system. These contradictory effects can be explained by two neuroreceptor sites that receive the neurotransmitters. Alcohol seems to have most direct effect on the GABA receptors. GABA is the major inhibitory neurotransmitter in the body and is ubiquitous in the brain. Thus alcohol has an inhibitory effect on the brain. Glutamate is the major excitatory neurotransmitter, and has the opposite effect of GABA. Recent evidence suggests that alcohol also acts on a form of glutamate receptors known as the NMDA receptors (T. Robinson, personal communication, 1991). Thus alcohol can produce both excitatory and inhibitory effects. (See discussion of neurotransmitters and the synapse in Chapter 3.)

As a sedative hypnotic, alcohol is capable of producing tolerance (more alcohol is required to produce the same behavioral effect over time) and physical dependence (withdrawal symptoms may be seen if high doses over time are discontinued or lowered). Alcohol may also produce psychological dependence (nonphysical symptoms on withdrawal characterized as intense craving for a substance which the user thinks is necessary for well-being). These aspects of alcohol and the nature of addiction are discussed further in Chapter 1.

Effects on the Fetus

The fetus has an immature liver that is unable to metabolize alcohol as it is metabolized in the adult. As the fetus excretes alcohol into the amniotic fluid, it is ingested again by the fetus; concentrations in the amniotic sac may be much higher than in the mother, and the alcohol will be metabolized to acetaldyhyde less efficiently. Blood alcohol levels remain high for twice as long in the fetus as in the mother.

Alcohol is known to be a contributor to low birth weight in the newborn, but other substances, such as smoking, can have the same effect. What accounts for the distinctive pattern of dysmorphic features and behaviors in FAS and FAE? Alcohol, like cocaine, can have direct and indirect effects on the fetus. The precise mechanism of alcohol's action on the fetus remains unknown, but there are several probable effects (Phillips et al., 1989). The hypotheses are based mostly on animal studies in which it is possible to experimentally control the quantity, duration, and timing of alcohol exposure. Data for humans are scant.

As in Chapter 3, a diagram depicts the direct and indirect effects. Direct effects do not depend on the mother, that is, the effects of alcohol act directly on the fetus. Indirect effects are the effects of alcohol on the mother that, in turn, compromise the fetus.

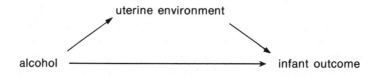

Direct Effects

Alcohol and acetaldehyde, the primary metabolite of alcohol, are the main teratogenic agents. They most likely interfere with protein synthesis in the fetal cells.

Indirect Effects

Maternal alcoholism may be accompanied by poor nutrition. Decreased availability of nutrients to the fetus could be due to poor maternal intake, decreased intestinal absorption of nutrients, impaired placental transfer, and/or deranged fetal utilization of selected foods (Fisher, 1988). However, the pattern of malformation associated with FAS has not been recognized in children born to undernourished women (Smith, 1947), in whom the offspring typically show catch-up growth not seen with FAS. Phillips et al. (1989) conclude that malnutrition is not essential to FAS but could compound its effect. They note, however, that there also is evidence that transfer of glucose, various amino acids, and zinc by the placenta may be impaired by ethanol intake, especially when ingested chronically.

Compromised blood flow to the placenta and fetus (hypoxia) is another possible explanation for the pathogenesis of FAS or FAE. Several studies suggest a direct constrictive effect of alcohol on umbilical vessels. Ethanol could restrict the flow of oxygen or valuable nutrients or both to the fetus.

Behaviors in Alcohol-Related Disorders

It is the neurobehaviors that are the most devastating to children and adults with FAS and FAE, and it is these that require the services of clinicians, educators, and health care providers. Some common behaviors observed in children, adolescents, and adults are summarized in Table 5–1. Of note is "indiscriminate attachment," which refers to the uncommon friendliness to people in the child's environment who are strangers

Table 5–1
Common characteristics of children and
adolescents with alcohol-related disorders

Hyperactive and distractible

Poor attention

Delayed motor development

Poor fine motor development

Learning problems

Uninhibited behavior

Socially engaging — but poor social skills

Indiscriminant attachment

Can be depressed and withdrawn

Poor judgment; do not learn from past experience

Source: Adapted from Streissguth et al. (1988, 1990).

or to whom friendly behavior would not be expected. Children with alcohol-related disorders are known to seek bodily contact — snuggling and hugging — when such behavior is not appropriate. Behaviors specific to age are discussed later in this chapter.

Common School-Related Behaviors

Individuals with alcohol-related disorders consistently do better in performance tasks — the more concrete the task, the better the performance — than in verbal tasks (Table 5–2). They also have poor verbal comprehension skills, despite their often comfortable, chatty manner. Their poor memory and attention present serious problems in their ability to adapt and attain functional skills.

Reading comprehension is poorer than word recognition, and this gap increases with age. The ability to generalize knowledge, both with language and numbers, requires a higher level of abstraction that many find difficult.

As with reading, there is no consistent pattern of spelling improvement noted with increasing age. However, particularly with girls, careful penmanship and relatively good spelling skills give the impression that they will be more functional than they actually are.

Arithmetic is the most difficult academic subject for children with alcohol-related disorders. Poor arithmetic skills present a major obstacle

Table 5–2
Common school behaviors in children and adolescents with alcohol-related disorders

Problems	Normal or Near Normal
Verbal comprehension	Verbal facility
Social adaptation	Cognition
Arithmetic	Reading and writing
Attention and memory	Expectation
Judgment	Aspirations
Abstract thinking	Performance on concrete tasks
Reading comprehension	Word recognition
Receptive vocabulary	Spelling

Source: Adapted from Streissguth et al. (1988, 1990).

to independent living, as many adults have trouble making change at the store and managing their finances. Poor arithmetic scores also reflect poor memory, poor abstract thinking, and difficulty with basic problem solving.

◼️ SCHOOL SERVICES

Importance of Diagnosis

The child with symptoms of FAS or FAE in a school caseload presents a diagnostic problem if the child does not exhibit developmental delay sufficient to qualify for service, but service is clearly needed. FAE children in particular may not have test scores that fall within the guidelines for severe language delay, yet they are distractible and have poor pragmatic skills. Under the guidelines for P.L. 94-142 and P.L. 99-457, they may qualify for services in some states, even in the absence of severely low test scores, if the at-risk condition of fetal alcohol exposure is included in the eligibility criteria. It may become the responsibility of any provider, in collaboration with others in the school system, to establish FAS or FAE as an etiology and thus enable children to meet eligibility criteria.

Children with alcohol-related problems are not often diagnosed in the schools for a number of reasons (Streissguth & Randels, 1988): First, most children with FAS are not raised by their biological mothers; therefore, maternal alcoholism as the cause of their disability often goes unnoticed in the community. Second, the milder cases may go undiagnosed because the physical characteristics are subtle, and central nervous system effects are often undifferentiating. Such children are found among the mildly disabled, often labeled as attention deficit disordered, speech and language handicapped, learning disabled, or not labeled at all. The link between the etiology of their disorder and their mother's drinking breaks down with each succeeding year following birth; an adolescent is even less likely to receive intervention on the basis of FAS/FAE than is a preschool or elementary school child.

Referral for Diagnosis

Diagnosis can be made by a pediatrician with an interest in dysmorphology or by referral to a *genetics clinic.* Genetics clinics can be found by calling the local chapter of the March of Dimes, which often sponsors such clinics. Visits are usually free, are covered by insurance, or have a sliding fee scale. It is not necessary to have a physician refer a patient. Schools may refer and parents may self-refer.

The following sections examine ways to investigate and document the two criteria for FAS/FAE — phenotype and prenatal alcohol exposure — and then to make a referral to the genetics clinic for diagnosis. Documenting the phenotype starts with assessment. Documenting alcohol exposure requires an alcohol history; it is often difficult and *not* essential to making a referral, although it is helpful.

Assessment

Assessment has two goals (assessment for determining therapy goals is excluded here): (1) Alcohol-related disorder is suspected and the information will be used for the goal of establishing the diagnosis; and (2) the child has been diagnosed as having an alcohol-related disorder, and appropriate placement or eligibility for service delivery is the goal.

Assessment, as with any disorder, will depend on the age of the child and the testing required by the school to certify eligibility for service or placement in special education. Tests should be *norm-referenced* to compare a child to peers in order to certify for service. Children with alcohol-related disorders generally have short attention spans and their activity levels will not permit protracted testing, particularly in younger children. Providers who work with infants and toddlers under the guidelines of P.L. 99-457, in which family assessment and family involvement are mandated, have the advantage of an assessment team. Those working with adolescents may not have a team, but collaboration with a social worker and/or school psychologist in addition to the classroom teacher should occur whenever possible. Assessment should include the following areas:

- ■ *Physical features.* Particular attention should be paid to oral-motor structure and function.
- ■ *Intellectual level.* A full-scale psychological evaluation should be done when the child enters school, or when the child comes to the attention of the evaluation team. The information is useful for comparison at key transition periods: preschool to elementary school, elementary school to middle school, middle school to high school.
- ■ *Achievement tests.* Levels of achievement in reading comprehension versus word recognition, arithmetic skills, and spelling.

- *Articulation test and language tests.* Receptive versus expressive language, language sampling or discourse analysis. Pay particular attention to sequencing in storytelling, in following directions, and to pragmatics.
- *Audiologic evaluation.* Every child at-risk for communication disorders should have an audiological evaluation. Treatment for otitis media or sensorineural hearing loss may be indicated.
- *Socialization and adaptation.* The Vineland Adaptive Behavior Scales (Sparrow, Balla, & Cicchetti, 1984) are recommended. The scales include four domains of behavior (Socialization, Communication, Motor Skills, and Daily Living Skills) and yield a score for each domain. The Socialization Scale, which encompasses interpersonal relationships, play and leisure time, and coping skills, is the most important of the scales if time is short. In addition, it is important to allow caregivers to relate behaviors that they perceive as problematic.
- *Family assessment.* Children with alcohol-related disorders live with either their family of origin or an adoptive or foster family. In the former, they are frequently raised in high-risk environments by mothers who continue to drink or struggle for sobriety and have few resources and little support. Thus, children with alcohol-related disorders are at a higher than average risk for physical abuse, sexual abuse, and neglect (Giunta & Streissguth, 1988). In the adoptive or foster care families, parents may have more stability and more resources, but are baffled by the child's behavior, whether or not they knew of the alcohol exposure when they took the child. If an assessment is done under P.L. 99-457 guidelines, a family assessment is mandatory, and many teams will have an assessment instrument. The *Family Needs Survey* (Bailey & Simeonsson, 1988) is highly recommended. It has a closed-end format: a checklist for needs in the areas of information, support, explaining to others, community services, financial help, and family functioning assistance. I ask the mother and father to fill it out without consulting with each other, then to turn it over and write down the three most important needs that they have with this child; those needs may not be mentioned on the checklist. Feelings such as fear that they may become so frustrated that they will abuse the child are much more likely to come to light in the open-end activity. The information can be used for the IFSP for family needs and strengths. It must be noted that school personnel have the re-

sponsibility to report all suspected child abuse to Child Protective Services.

Taking an Alcohol History

The most important point to be made in this section is that school personnel need not have an alcohol history in order to make a referral for suspected alcohol-related disorder. Finding confirming information can be a real problem for school providers for several reasons.

- Alcohol exposure makes us all uncomfortable. We would like to believe that it does not happen. We all have emotional baggage when it comes to alcohol use.
- Obtaining an alcohol history may be impossible because the child is in foster care or has been adopted and birth history is unknown, or because the birth mother is uncooperative.
- We fear that to ask a mother about alcohol use is an invasion of her privacy and we worry about privacy laws and our liability.

An illustration of our unease is the following. Some materials are available with the stated purpose of helping health care professionals learn to take an alcohol history. One of these, "Taking a Drinking History" (see Appendix B), is a short videotape dramatization of a health provider taking a history from a pregnant woman. According to Weiner, Rosett, and Mason (1985), its purpose is:

> to evoke discussion about attitudes toward the patient. It illustrates a difficult and resistant woman from whom information on alcohol is successfully obtained . . . In the film, the counselor clarifies vague responses, trying to determine precisely what the patient's drinking patterns are. Acceptance of evasive answers can reinforce the patient's denial. By mentioning large amounts of alcohol, the counselor acknowledges that the patient is drinking heavily and thereby facilitates reporting high intake levels. Although the interview is discomforting and the patient is stressed, she continues to answer questions.
>
> A therapeutic alliance is developed in the film. The counselor sustains empathic attitudes and avoids angry confrontation. She is objective and nonmoralistic, allowing the patient to report drinking at any level. Her persistent questions provide information not only on quantity consumed but also on circumstances surrounding use. Counselor and patient are both made aware of the drinking pattern. (p. 35)

"Jane" is asked when and how much she drinks of first beer, then wine, then spirits. In each case she at first denies that she drinks "much" or that she even enjoys drinking but that she does it to go along with her husband and loosen up at parties. Under questioning Jane is found to imbibe considerable amounts of alcohol in a week's time. She is then cautioned about her drinking and told that drinking during her pregnancy may harm her baby. Portions of the dialogue are presented below (Weiner et al., 1985).

Counselor: Okay Jane, we've gone over your health history and your nutrition and your eating habits. Now I need to get some lifestyle information from you. Okay. How about alcohol; do you drink beer?

Jane: I drink beer on weekends.

Counselor: How many cans of beer at a time?

Jane: I don't know. I don't count them.

Counselor: On an average weekend. Let's think back to this past weekend. How many beers did you have?

Jane: Um. Friday. We buy a case on Friday for the weekend.

Counselor: And how long did that last?

Jane: Say, this weekend, ah, it took us through the weekend.

Counselor: Weekdays?

Jane: I don't drink during the week.

Counselor: Do you drink any beer at all on weekdays?

Jane: Well, um . . . couple watching TV, you know. That's, I don't really, I'm not drinking during the week. Just a couple of beers.

Counselor: So two cans while watching TV on a weekday? Do you ever drink more than that?

Jane: No, no.

Counselor: Okay, what about wine, do you drink wine? (p. 33)

I have shown this videotape to graduate classes for several years, and the reaction has become predictable. A majority of the class reacts to the counselor as unduly intrusive; they report that she should not have asked the questions in the way that she did and that she made Jane defensive and alarmed. Others in the class think that the questions were appropriate but that the counselor was "cold," "judgmental," and "unfeeling" toward Jane. The class uniformly reports that the questioning made them uncomfortable. When asked how the counselor could have gotten the information without direct questioning, few alternatives could be given. It seems that the stated purpose was not achieved.

This experience produced considerable unease in speech-language pathologists, who until that time did not have to consider taking a drinking history as part of their scope of practice. We do not want to ask questions that we never expected to have to ask. The farther we get away from our traditional base, the more likely we are to feel uncomfortable. The truth is, however, that very few professionals in the health or education fields, with the exception of those in addiction treatment, are comfortable with this kind of questioning.

DIRECT QUESTIONING. Methods are available to ask questions in a routine fashion. The very simplest diagnostic tool possessed by all providers is the case history form. The routine history-taking process affords the provider the easiest entry into the subject of alcohol intake during pregnancy. Information on maternal drinking history should be routinely asked in the workup of patients of any age with developmental disabilities, attentional defects, and/or conduct disorders (Streissguth et al., 1991). However, many clinics and schools do not even include direct questions concerning alcohol on the case history forms; if it is included, there may be a blank by the word "alcohol" as there is by "smoking," which leaves the provider at a loss as to how to approach the subject. Questions about alcohol use should be consistent with other questions in the history form. It is preferable not to ask, "Do you drink?" This question connotes problem drinking and usually will get a negative response. Also, "You didn't drink, did you?" suggests a negative reply and will yield little information. The preferred method is to say, "How much did you smoke when you were pregnant with George? How much did you drink?" Given any answer other than abstinence, you can follow up with, "How many drinks did you have at one time?" Pursue the answers until a profile is given. Then confirm the answers: "Am I correct that you drank vodka on weekends only and that you had about 6 drinks on weekend nights in about the first 3 months of your pregnancy?"

In summary, get a drinking history if you can. If you cannot, leave it to the professionals at the genetics clinic. It is more important for you to make the referral than to have a positive drinking history.

Referral Process

After you have done your assessment of the child and gathered pertinent information from the caregiver, you are ready to make the referral. The following are suggested steps for that process.

- Inform your supervisor of the problem and your suspected diagnosis of FAS or FAE.
- Call the closest genetics clinic and speak to a counselor about the procedure for your referral to *rule out alcohol-related anomalies*. Ask the counselor what the parents should expect when they visit as to time involved, who should go along, and costs.
- Gather information from the classroom teacher and/or team regarding the diagnosis. (See the tables of behaviors, Tables 5–3, 5–4, and 5–5 in the following sections.) Synthesize the information. You will need to send it to the genetics clinic before the visit.
- Approach the mother or caregiver. It could occur at an IFSP meeting, an IEPC, or as a private conversation. The conversation may be something like the following.

"Mrs. Smith, George seems to need help to concentrate on his work and with his language activities at school and there are some things that I'm puzzled about. Have you ever had him evaluated by anyone other than here at school?"

The question at the end is specific and can be repeated if it is not answered. Any other consultations should be entered into the child's record. You can then follow up by asking what was learned at those consultations. Did the evaluator have a reason or cause for the behaviors that you are seeing? Is the caregiver satisfied that everything is now known that could be known?

"There is a resource that could be very helpful to us here at school that I would like you to consider. There is a team of specialists at the (hospital or other site of the genetics clinic) that specializes in diagnosing children's problems that probably started at birth. It's a genetics clinic. I have the phone number and the name of the person you should talk to. If you would like, I can make the call for you for an appointment."

The information you have about the procedures of the clinic should also be given at this time. Caregivers should be told that, even though a diagnosis might be troubling, it will enable us to better help the child. Offer to go along as a history source.

- Have the caregiver sign a release form giving you permission to send copies of school assessments to the genetics clinic.

■ Send a cover letter to the clinic explaining why the referral was made along with information that is pertinent. The genetics clinic will send a report to you as the referral source.

Caregiver Reactions

Reactions to such a request are as varied as the caregivers' personalities. It is possible that parents, particularly foster and adoptive parents, will welcome the opportunity to receive some help, particularly if it means they can now obtain suitable programs for their child. It is also possible that they will ignore your request out of fear and denial. Dorris (1989) related how he, as an adoptive parent, denied his son's school difficulties; it was the fault of his start in life, the school, the teachers, anything but the possibility that something could be wrong with his son. If alcohol is a problem in the home, denial is a fact of daily life. If you have planned carefully for this referral, and if you have the backing of team members and the administration, your united front will make the request more difficult to ignore.

■□ AGE-SPECIFIC BEHAVIORS

There is considerable variability in the physical, academic, and behavioral characteristics of individuals with alcohol-related disorder. In the following sections, common characteristics, derived from averaging across individuals with a wide spectrum of abilities, will be summarized with the caution that individual children may vary from these patterns. For example, microcephaly is found in most FAS children and adults, but individuals with the diagnosis of FAS have been found who have normal head circumference. The profiles are based on the best research to date (Streissguth et al., 1988; Streissguth et al., 1991). Some of the studies included only Native American subjects, but the types of deficits seen are similar regardless of race, sex, age, residential location, IQ score, or amount of education. Many of the subjects were not retarded and did not qualify for special education.

Infancy

At birth, these babies are often tremulous and irritable, have a weak sucking reflex, and hypotonia. They also fail to tune out intrusive stimuli and involuntarily respond to noises and other environmental stimuli (lack of habituation). It is also usual for them to be readmitted to the hospital during the first few months of life for failure to thrive, pneumonia, and evaluation of heart defects, hip dysplasia, and developmental delay. Feeding difficulties are a concern to caretakers during this period. Sleep patterns may be erratic, with poor differentiation of sleep/wake cycles.

An infant and his or her caregiver(s) are part of a system of interaction. They affect each other mutually, in complex ways (Clark & Sparks, 1988). A healthy infant is born with an amazing capacity to engage adults and communicate needs, but most important, to make that adult fall in love with it. The demanding behaviors characteristic of infants and young children with FAS and FAE (see Table 5–3) make these children difficult to care for, even for the most capable and patient parents. Such a child placed with an alcoholic mother poses a double jeopardy. Despite good intentions, such mothers have difficulty providing the calm, nurturing, structured, consistent environment that appears to be most facilitating to the optimal development of children with alcohol-related disorder. At best the behaviors can lead to poor bonding and attachment and a negative climate for communication development; at worst, the situation can lead to abuse. (For more about the alcoholic mother, see Chapter 1.)

Table 5–3
Common behaviors of infancy and early childhood in alcohol-related disorders

Poor habituation

Sleep disturbances

Poor sleep/wake cycle

Poor sucking response

Failure to thrive

Distractibility/hyperactivity

Delays in walking/talking

Delays in toilet training

Difficulty following directions

Temper tantrums/disobedience

Prone to otitis media

Source: Adapted from Streissguth et al. (1988, 1990).

Older infants are often described as "very good." They are usually very oriented toward people and often show no stranger anxiety.

Language, Speech, and Oral-Motor Development

As the infants get older, they may be slow to master motor milestones, slow to start to say words, and slow to combine words. Adjusting to solid food is often difficult, and caregivers continue to complain of poor appetites and disinterest in food.

Early Childhood

During this period, children with FAS are usually short and elf-like in manner and appearance. They flit from one thing to another, moving with "butterfly-like" movements. They seem alert, outgoing, excessively friendly, and more interested in people than objects. Their needs for bodily contact often seem insatiable; they like to touch, fondle, pat, and kiss and usually have a happy disposition. However, they can be stubborn and unyielding in their demands.

Hyperactivity is most pronounced during these years. At home they may be "into everything," and their first preschool experience is often difficult because they "can't sit still a minute." They also are often fearless and do not respond well to verbal restrictions. They tend to wander away, go into the street, and need closer supervision than other children. Problems with coordination, fine motor control, and gross motor control become apparent as they try to draw and to ride a tricycle.

Many caregivers find these children endearing during this period, and their slow development and poor performance are often excused on the basis of their small size. "He'll outgrow it" is a commonly expressed hope at this age, and developmental delays are often not taken seriously by the family. However, children with serious hyperactivity are usually diagnosed at this age. Alert preschool and Headstart teachers are often the first to recommend a diagnostic evaluation.

Language, Speech, and Oral-Motor Development

Language development is often delayed, but seems to be less of a problem to parents because they tend to adjust their expectations in accordance with the children's small size. As speech emerges, articulation defects, echolalia, and perseveration are often noted, along with a shortness of sentences. Receptive language seems to be less of a problem than language expression.

Early School Years

When the child with an alcohol-related disorder must utilize higher cognitive processes to meet academic demands in a classroom situation, hyperactivity, learning problems, and difficulties with classroom management may become apparent (Table 5–4). These behaviors may occur in children of normal or near normal intelligence. Gold and Sherry (1984) reported studies of such children in which those with less severe hyperactivity were distractible, had short attention spans, and could be described as "fidgety." Streissguth, Herman, and Smith (1978) described the children as "always on the go," and "never sits still." In addition, inability to function without intense one-to-one or small group instruction was uniformly found in the population studied by Shaywitz, Cohen, and Shaywitz (1980). Comments such as "behind ever since he entered school," "an itch," "easily distracted," "never concentrates unless directly supervised by a teacher," "seems to have the skills yet is not learning" were noted in all of these children's records. All were recommended for special services by the third grade.

Referral for special education occurs during this stage for the most obviously mentally handicapped children with FAS, and they usually continue in a special classroom or school during the rest of their school years. However, the less handicapped children with FAS often continue in regular classrooms during their early school years. Reading and writing skills during the first 2 years may not be noticeably delayed, particularly for children who have repeated kindergarten and are not hyperactive. When one compares their achievement test scores to their

Table 5–4
Common behaviors in the early school years in alcohol-related disorders

Delayed physical and cognitive development (speech)
Hyperactivity, memory deficit, and impulsivity
Poor comprehension of social rules and expectations
Easily influenced and unable to understand consequences
Give appearance of ability due to apparent verbal skills without actual capabilities
Temper tantrums, lying, stealing, disobedience, and defiance of authority

Source: Adapted from Streissguth et al. (1988, 1990).

IQ test scores at this age, they may appear to be achieving quite well relative to their IQ scores.

Attentional deficits become more manifest during the early school years as the demands for classroom attention increase. Emotional lability is also more pronounced at this time, and poor impulse control, memory deficits, and social intrusiveness are also observed. A well-done study by Streissguth, Barr, Sampson, Parrish-Johnson, Kirchner, and Martin (1986) is one of the few in which the mothers were primarily white, married, and middle-class. The large sample of children with FAS and control subjects were between 6½ to 8½ years old. The study addressed attentional deficits in school-age children exposed prenatally to alcohol. Prenatal alcohol exposure was significantly related to attentional deficits and reaction time in the FAS children. The children were not tested under classroom conditions, but given the levels of distractibility the authors found in the FAS children, it could be inferred that they would show even greater problems with distractibilty if tested in a group setting. Poor peer relations and social isolation may be noted in the more functional children. Excessive demands for bodily contact often continue during this period, and interest in sexual exploration with other children may get them into trouble. Hostility and destructiveness are sometimes seen, but appear to be related to the living situation (current or previous) rather than a typical manifestation of FAS per se.

Language, Speech, and Oral-Motor Development

Expressive language may be delayed. Children with alcohol-related disorders often lack richness of speech, thought, and grammatical complexity. They are often excessively talkative and intrusive, for example, asking a lot of questions, which gives the superficial appearance that speech is not impaired (Streissguth et al., 1988).

One of the few studies by speech-language pathologists is by Becker, Warr-Leeper, and Leeper (1990). Their study of a small matched cohort of FAS and non-FAS Native American children ages 4½ to 9½ years old and matched for foster family living environments, points up the striking incidence of deviations of structure and function exhibited in the speech mechanisms of FAS and control subjects. The FAS group showed a higher percentage of deviations in the structure of the dentition and the gingiva, as well as in functional movement of the tongue and larynx. The authors examined not only the so-called oral-peripheral mechanism, but eight major valves along the vocal tract, and the FAS group demonstrated deficiencies in one or more of these valves.

Transitional Periods

Two critical school periods for these children are the transitions between elementary and middle school and between middle and upper school. Decreased adult supervision, increasing peer pressure, and increasing academic demands appear to be the key features. There is increased truancy, school refusals, and school dropouts at both these transitional points, as well as an increase in behavioral disruption in the classroom. All of these behaviors should be viewed as symptomatic of the need to reevaluate the classroom placement and educational expectations of these children. An appropriate topic for the Individual Educational Planning Committee (IEPC) meeting is collaboration between home and all school personnel for consistent and immediate discipline.

Middle and High School Years

School achievement usually reaches the maximum point at about grades 6 to 8, with reading and spelling often being superior to arithmetic skills (Table 5-5; see also Table 5-2.) Increased difficulties maintaining attention, completing assignments, and mastering new academic skills converge to make school attendance increasingly stressful. However, good verbal facility, a superficially friendly social manner, and good intentions often continue to mask the seriousness of the situation. Increased stress and decreased classroom satisfaction can lead to lack of motivation and poor school attendance during this period, particularly for children without a strong and supportive family. They are at risk for increased truancy and school drop-out. This is of particular concern because their low adaptive living skills and poor intellectual development do not make them good candidates for employment or independent living. Concerns of parents and teachers include difficulty staying on task, distracting other children, poor use of language, inability to structure their work time, and a constant need for monitoring and attention. Stubbornness, immaturity, poor self-image, poor social attitude, a need for constant supervision, and difficulty dealing with change are frequently described problems. Preparing for the world of work has its own problems in that these individuals do not do well with repetitive work tasks, particularly when left unsupervised. They are people-oriented and will walk away from a boring task.

Impulsiveness, lack of inhibition, and naivete are common among individuals with alcohol-related disorders, and these attributes are complicated by the physical maturity of an adolescent or adult. Concerns

Table 5-5

Common characteristics of adolescents with
alcohol-related disorders

Reach academic ceiling

Sexual difficulties (easily exploited, inappropriate
sexual behavior)

Depression, social isolation

Pregnancy/fathering

Truancy and school dropout

Pragmatic language problems

Naive, childlike manner

Very poor judgment

Attention deficits, restless, move from place to place

Arithmetic disability — worse than reading

Memory problems, especially visual spatial

Difficulty abstracting and seeing cause and effect

Poor impulse control

Disoriented time and space

Source: Adapted from Streissguth et al. (1988, 1990).

about inappropriate sexual activity begin to surface once the children
reach the age of 10 or 11 years, particularly after the age of 12. Female
adolescents are often seen as passive, acquiescent, and easily victimized.
The fear of sexual victimization is a real one, as their excessive curiosity,
interest in tactile contact, impulsivity, and poor judgment often place
them in potentially exploitive circumstances. They have difficulty com-
prehending social situations, remembering the appropriate behavior,
and knowing when to say "no."

Language, Speech, and Oral-Motor Development

Adolescents and adults with alcohol-related disabilities are noted to
have a range of communication problems that are commonly found in
conjunction with intellectual impairment and to have some other deficits
that appear to be distinctive, if not unique. In the former category are
receptive difficulties — inability to listen to a story — and expressive
language problems — inability to relate an experience in detail or give
detailed directions to others. These problems are to be expected in indi-

viduals who have difficulty with abstraction and memory. Articulation problems are not notably more numerous at this age. However, they do have significant problems with dentition and malocclusion that can interfere with articulation.

The most distinctive problem for these individuals is that they are so superficially talkative that people expect them to be more competent cognitively and behaviorally than they are. They are noted to talk too much and too fast with little to say. Furthermore, pragmatics (interrupting or poor timing, using inappropriate conversational topics, and dwelling on one particular subject) are a problem regardless of intellectual level. The pragmatic problems are consistent with difficulty in remembering social rules and picking up on social cues.

Body language remains a problem in adolescence: there is little sense of personal space, and the individuals are very "touchy" and have inappropriate and excessive curiosity. Such behavior is a barrier to making friends, although most of the individuals are described as having a "sweet" disposition.

Speech problems seen in the more handicapped individuals include perseveration in written and spoken language, echolalia, and the repetitive use of words or phrases. Some have been reported to repeat nonsense sounds or carry on nonsensical conversations when no one was around.

■□ SUMMARY

In this chapter we have examined a considerable body of research that led to outlining the characteristics of individuals with alcohol-related disorders, from infancy to adulthood. We have also discussed the role of the provider in diagnosis and referral in collaboration with other school personnel, keeping in mind that school personnel can identify but not diagnose FAS or FAE. In the following chapter, this information will be translated into guidelines for intervention strategies.

Interventions for Alcohol-Related Disorders

■□ **FETAL ALCOHOL SYNDROME**

Melinda's Story

Melinda's birthweight was 3 lbs 14 oz. Her mother, age 34 at Melinda's birth, was hit by a car during her pregnancy, when she was binge drinking. She also had a couple of grand mal seizures while intoxicated during her pregnancy. She left the home 3 days after Melinda's birth and died of alcoholism when Melinda was 5 years old. Melinda was raised as the only child of her father, who was noted throughout her school history as being overprotective and uncooperative with school personnel. She crept at 9 months, sat at 14 months, and walked at 18 months. She used a few single words at 18 months.

Melinda's father brought her to our clinic for a speech and language evaluation when she was 2½ years old. She weighed only 15 lbs and was 31 inches tall. She had clefts of the hard and soft palate, mild to moderate

conductive hearing loss, chronic serous otitis media with surgical placement of tubes to allow for continuous drainage from the middle ear, ventricular septal defect which closed spontaneously, significant hand trem-
or, and vision problems. To demonstrate her language ability, she and
her father ran through a series of well-rehearsed "tricks," for example,
Where's your nose? Cover your eyes. Melinda had no evident spontaneous language. She was very friendly and not at all fearful of the testing situation but she was not responsive to normative testing. My
recommendations for Melinda at age 2½ were:

1. Improve her hearing status. Refer her for reevaluation of her
   drainage tubes or hearing aids.
2. Give her intensive daily speech and language therapy in a program for the hearing impaired in the school district.
3. Refer her to an oral cleft team.

Melinda was fitted for hearing aids and glasses, and she wore
neither. She was placed in a program for the hearing impaired where she
would have daily speech and language stimulation, but her father
removed her after a few days because he felt she was not properly supervised, and she might get hurt. She received speech therapy at various
community clinics in her preschool years, but her attendance was extremely inconsistent. At age 9 she was 45 inches tall and weighed 38 lbs.
A second set of upper central incisors erupted, which resulted in considerable dental crowding. She had surgeries for closure of hard and soft
palates and removal of ventilation tubes bilaterally when she was 9 years
old. Follow-up evaluation showed a 10 dB conductive hearing loss in
both ears, improved from a 20–30 dB loss before surgery. She was
known to be friendly, sweet, and sociable throughout her life. Her father
described Melinda as well above average in intelligence and described
her marks in school as high, with no low grades. Placement in a learning
disabled class was recommended when she began school, but her father
insisted that she be placed in regular education. She did receive speech
therapy for language and articulation. At age 9 she was in the 2nd percentile on the Peabody Picture Vocabulary Test. At age 11 she was 1 standard deviation below the mean for language and thus qualified for
language therapy. The next year she did not qualify for language services, but she received therapy for articulation. When she was in eighth
grade she was dismissed from therapy because she had met the speech
goals and was intelligible "within her limitations." At age 16 she is still
very small. She has friends at school and is liked by her teachers. She is a
C and D student but is hanging on in school. One teacher noted that she

could not remember the combination for the lock on her locker, so she leaves it unlocked.

Melinda was known to have FAS during her school years. She demonstrated diagnostic features in all three criteria: growth deficiency, dysmorphology that included cleft lip and palate, and neurobehaviors that included her hand tremor and learning difficulties. However, as so often happens, her speech problems were attributed to her cleft palate and to her hearing loss. Although those problems certainly needed intervention, she was not eligible for speech and language intervention on the basis of her FAS status with its attendant risk for language development. She does not exhibit challenging behaviors and her academic difficulties are easy to ignore. There is no special help available in her high school to develop vocational skills. The speech and language therapy that she received was traditional; its focus was on articulation and syntax rather than on pragmatic skills necessary to find and keep a job. Her father is still in control of her life, and chances for her to live independently after graduation are questionable.

■□ FETAL ALCOHOL EFFECT

Danny's Story

Danny was adopted at age 6 months, the first of his parents' two adopted boys. His parents were told that his birth mother drank "moderately" during the first 3 months of her pregnancy and then stopped drinking. At birth he weighed 8 lb 5 oz and was 19 in. long. He had tetralogy of Fallot, a heart condition, and bilateral club feet that required casting for a year and special shoes after that. Open heart surgery corrected the heart defect at 13 months. When Danny was 3½, he was not toilet trained and his speech was unintelligible. His pediatrician referred him to his school district where he was carefully evaluated by a multidisciplinary team: occupational therapy, physical therapy, and a teacher of the preprimary impaired classroom. The latter evaluation was done in the home. They agreed that Danny was developing normally in all areas with the exception of communication skills (borderline) and academic skills (significant). Placement in the preprimary impaired classroom was recommended at the Individualized Educational Planning Committee meeting.

Danny's mother brought him to our clinic the next week for an evaluation. Danny relied heavily on vowels for communication, which he delivered with various intonation; he omitted nearly all initial consonants.

We obtained a language sample for expressive language evaluation (he rarely used both subject and verb) and the Sequenced Inventory of Communication Development (Hedrick, Prather, & Tobin, 1984) for receptive language. His hearing status was normal. Danny's parents elected to have him attend the university clinic rather than follow the school's recommendation. He made rapid progress in articulation and language goals in one-to-one therapy, with each of three clinicians noting his high resistance to therapy. His mother attributed his apparent unhappiness to his father's absence from the home on business trips. He was dismissed from therapy a year later when his speech and language skills were within normal limits, and he had reached a plateau in his progress.

Danny is now 7 years old (weight and height are at the 40th percentile) and he has never been in public school; his mother teaches him at home and reports that he is progressing very well in reading and math. She describes him as developmentally on track in all areas except emotional development; he throws temper tantrums when he is unable to do something well. She describes it as being "out of control." He participates in church activities, a bowling league, and takes piano lessons. He is beginning to control his temper, and when his parents feel that the temper can be handled in school, they will send him, probably to a Christian parochial school.

Danny was not diagnosed as having FAE, and that diagnosis would be difficult and ambiguous. He does not exhibit growth disorder. Dysmorphology is questionable and would be a clinical decision; he appeared to have short palpebral fissures and flat philtrum (see Chapter 5). Any neurobehavioral aberrations at birth are unknown to his adoptive parents. He exhibits challenging behaviors now, but certainly children who are not exposed prenatally to alcohol also have temper tantrums. Danny's behavior does seem to be unusual; his parents think he needs more supervision than he could get in school in order to stay in control. It is this pattern of symptoms with the mother's positive alcohol history that points to FAE.

◼️ INFERENCE FROM RESEARCH

Although the research for describing the characteristics of those with alcohol-related disabilities provides a substantial knowledge base, there is little information on interventions for FAS and FAE that is based on solid program evaluation. Most of the intervention literature is based on experience and efficacy for children and adults with similar behaviors rather than reports of interventions based on research in alcohol-related disorders. There are no curricula for FAS children, nor should there be, as their needs and abilities are varied. In this chapter, the research conclusions from the previous chapter will serve as guidelines for structuring intervention strategies. The intervention strategies rely heavily on the work of Burgess and Streissguth (1990, 1992).

- Children with alcohol-related disorders are most often misdiagnosed in schools as having the following disorders: attention deficit disorder (ADD) because they have difficulty sustaining attention; receptive language disorders because they have low scores on standardized receptive language scales; and oppositional deviant disorders because they frequently lose their temper and seem out of control.
- The greatest communication problem in FAS and FAE is a marked discrepancy between seemingly high verbal skills and inability to communicate effectively. Their language skills often appear much greater than their actual ability to communicate effectively.
- The greatest problem for functioning appropriately in society is poor judgment. They cannot predict the consequences of their behavior.
- The greatest educational problem is poor attention. FAS children often have severe attentional deficits that interfere with school performance during the school-age years and work performance during adulthood.
- FAS and FAE individuals have lower academic achievement than is expected. They are often described as having "no common sense" and "not using what they have."
- FAE should not be viewed as less severe than FAS; the physical characteristics may not be present, but the neurobehavioral characteristics may be as severe as for FAS.
- Neurobehavioral effects of prenatal alcohol exposure, expressed as cognitive and behavioral differences in both FAS and FAE, are not transient effects. They should be seen as lifelong disorders.
- Adaptive skills can be more severely affected than would be expected from IQ and achievement test scores.
- Teachers find affected young students to be impulsive, have poor attention spans, and to have difficulty making transitions.
- Older affected individuals show impulsivity and unwillingness to stay with frustrating tasks.

- Inappropriate social behavior includes stealing, lying, and the potential to be exploited sexually.
- The combination of poor self-control and inadequate communication skills creates learning and social problems.
- Vocational skills are often poor; affected individuals become bored and distracted easily when doing repetitive tasks or when left unsupervised.
- Children and adults with alcohol-related disabilities are underserved by school programs because they are undetected and because FAS and FAE are not recognized as conditions that qualify for special services in the schools. They are often classified as learning disabled or emotionally disturbed when, in fact, their disabilities extend beyond those categorical boundaries.
- Individuals affected by alcohol-related disorders have great variability in communication skills, ranging from apparently normal language to no verbal communication at all.
- Deviations of the structure and function of the speech mechanism, including abnormalities in the major valves of the vocal tract, are common in individuals with FAS.
- Challenging behaviors can be viewed as forms of communication in FAS and FAE individuals.

▢ GUIDELINES FOR INTERVENTION STRATEGIES

Target Functional Skills

Make independence and productivity the goals of education and therapy so that when these children reach adulthood they are functioning as fully as they are able. To reach those goals, we must go beyond classroom boundaries and target functional skills to be used not only at school but in homes and communities. The content of functional skills curricula is different for small children than for high school students and must be adapted for those with varying cognitive abilities. For some children, "functional" may mean following traditional academic curricula. To be independent, they need to ride buses, prepare meals, and use money appropriately. To hold a job, they must learn the necessary skills to get the job but they must also have the social skills to keep that job. Interventions should be focused on both present and future environments in which students will live and work and should teach skills specific to those settings (Burgess & Streissguth, 1990).

Make Education Culturally Relevant

Educational programs must consider the cultural origin of children and prepare them to function in the environments in which they will live as adults. This is particularly true for Native Americans and Alaskan natives who have significantly high rates of alcohol-related disorders. Children with FAS and FAE should experience community values just as children in regular education do. Educational and therapy experiences can involve cultural experiences.

Use Nontraditional Therapy Approaches

Speech and language therapy must encompass all forms of communication: verbal, written, gestural, and behavioral skills that allow an individual to participate in a social environment. Providers must teach students with FAS and FAE to relate their needs to others, whether verbally or through other communication systems, in appropriate ways. Think of communication skills in the context of social skills instruction; the two are inseparable and essential sets of skills to live and work in the community. Small children can learn to communicate their needs, interact with peers, and respond to others appropriately. By high school, students should be learning more complex communication and social skills, such as how to interact with employers and co-workers, make and maintain friendships, and behave appropriately with friends of the opposite sex. The point cannot be overemphasized: Traditional speech therapy goals, such as using three new words in a sentence, are inappropriate. Functional goals, such as staying out of a stranger's car, are appropriate. The key concept is to focus on both present and future environments in which students will live and work and to teach skills specific to those settings.

Teach Students to Make Choices

It is crucial for providers and teachers to recognize that students with FAS or FAE, regardless of age or ability, may lack the skill of making choices. Burgess and Streissguth (1992) give the example of a child who works dilligently for free time, but when that time comes he wanders around the room bothering other children or getting in the way of their activities. That child may be communicating the fact that he has not learned how to choose an appropriate activity for free time. Making choices must be taught in a systematic fashion, beginning with a few concrete choices, then gradually becoming more abstract. Once he has been taught, the choice the child has made must be honored, or we will teach him that there is no meaning in his decision. For example, if a child refuses milk with his snack, we do not just give it to him anyway, we honor his choice. Give lots of opportunities to practice. Such skills may not be within the realm of typical educational programs, but they are critical to the survival of persons with alcohol-related disorders in the real world.

Emphasize Communication Skills in the Classroom

The first step in developing appropriate, effective communication skills is for teachers to learn to recognize and honor their students' communicative attempts, because without effective verbal language, students will find other ways to communicate their needs. Providers and teachers can collaborate to discover and interpret those communicative attempts. Watch facial expressions and body language as means of expression. A child with poor verbal skills may let a teacher know that she needs help by something as subtle as moving her paper aside or something as dramatic as tearing it. Recognizing such behaviors as communication and shaping them into appropriate language is an important part of a comprehensive program. For example, the provider who observes the communicative attempts with the paper can work to help the child recognize what she needs to communicate (asking for help) and how to communicate her message. The provider completes the therapy goal by telling the teacher what the new communication is and helping the teacher to reinforce the behavior (Burgess & Streissguth, 1990).

Make Learning Community-Based and Have Generalization as the Outcome

Teach students to generalize what they learn beyond the walls of the classroom or the school building. Provide students with FAS and FAE with opportunities to practice their new skills in real settings, for example, using money in the grocery store (Burgess & Streissguth, 1990). Providing practice is more appropriate for the provider than for the teacher because the provider can take as few as one or two students at a time on an "excursion." Use role-playing before the actual experience, with students in the group playing the different parts of customer, clerk, and check-out person. Work from that concrete experience to generalize to other customer-salesperson situations, for example, "We have learned how to buy something in a grocery store. Now, how do you buy something in a hardware store?" By the same token, help students to understand the consequences of their behavior, for example, "What happens if you take something that doesn't belong to you?" or "What happens if someone offers drugs to you and you take them?"

Listen to Parents

Providers can collaborate with teachers more easily than with parents in many cases. However, the input of parents is very important, even beyond the early intervention years. Parents can collaborate with the provider in setting goals that involve home social situations. The provider can then help the student with FAS or FAE to choose an appropriate behavior for the situation and provide practice through role-playing.

Manage Challenging Behaviors Through Communication

One of the most important breakthroughs in behavior management in recent years was the realization that inappropriate or "challenging" behaviors are a form of communication. This is particularly true for students with FAS and FAE who have difficulty with communication. When they cannot express their needs or feelings in socially acceptable ways, they may resort to behaviors that, although less acceptable to adults, get the desired effects. We may typically view problem behaviors as malicious or attention getting. In reality, a student may be trying to communicate any one of a thousand messages such as, "The work is too hard," "It's too easy," or "I have to go to the bathroom." The key for us is to look for communicative intent (Burgess & Streissguth, 1992).

To manage challenging behaviors, the first step is to generate hypotheses about the child's message. Again provider and teacher, perhaps with help from the parent, can collaborate to generate ideas. Once we have an idea of intention, we can test our hypothesis by choosing an alternative form of communication and teaching the student to use it. The alternative form can be as simple as helping her to verbalize what she is feeling (e.g., "I see by your behavior that you're telling me the work is too hard") or more complex (e.g., gestures, signs, alternative communication devices). The point is to help the student to learn a more appropriate way to communicate the message she was expressing through her behavior (Burgess & Streissguth, 1992).

To reduce challenging behaviors by teaching communication, it is worth repeating that it is essential to provide opportunities for the student to communicate and then to honor his attempts. Although time consuming at first, it is critical for him to build trust in the fact that his communication has meaning. Then we can slowly and systematically build delays by asking the child to wait before we honor his request.

Another important aspect of behavior management is to plan ahead. When we are in the heat of a crisis, we all need to "get control." That is exactly the opposite of the goal of intervention, which is to give students control of their own behavior so they can become independent. If we plan ahead, perhaps with a team or through collaboration, we can prepare for a challenging situation, and each person in the environment is more likely to behave consistently (Burgess & Streissguth, 1992).

For students with FAS and FAE, structure must be balanced with opportunities to practice independence. Although it is important to provide structure, it is equally important to give students opportunities to use the skills we have taught them. If we try to "control" young people when they are ready to grow, we can cause them to resort to challenging behaviors to meet their needs. In addition, if we keep a child's life too rigidly structured, she can never learn to manage herself. At 18 or 21, she will still be dependent on adults for all the decisions in her life (Burgess & Streissguth, 1992).

■□ AGE-SPECIFIC INTERVENTIONS

In this section, we move from general guidelines to interventions appropriate to various ages.

Interventions in Infancy and Early Childhood

Early diagnosis is desirable so that appropriate early interventions can prevent some disorders and ameliorate others (Table 6–1). However, according to Little, Snell, and Rosenfeld (1990), the prospect of general early identification of infants with FAS seems unlikely in light of a recent report from one of the largest obstetrical services in the United States, which documented a 100% failure rate in diagnosing FAS at delivery. After the diagnosis of FAS or FAE has been made, the spokesperson for the P.L. 99-457 team must undertake intervention with the birth or foster parents. Caretakers need to learn all they can about the signs, symptoms, medical, social, and behavioral consequences of alcohol-related disorders. This information is particularly important for birth mothers who are still drinking and at risk of having another affected child. Intervenors must be emphatic that mothers who are drinking must not breast-feed and that infants should not be given alcohol for colic or any other reason.

TABLE 6-1

Interventions in infancy and early childhood

Provide early diagnosis and intervention

Provide intervention with birth or foster parents

Provide education to parents regarding physical/psychological needs of affected infant/child

Provide careful monitoring of physical development and health

Assign service coordinator for coordinating services

Encourage preschool attendance

Encourage respite care for parents

Source: Adapted from Streissguth, et al. (1988, 1990).

Caregivers need to set realistic goals and expectations for their children and for themselves, particularly in the areas of academic and social functioning. Perhaps because of their verbal facility, children with alcohol-related disorders are often thought, on casual observation, to be brighter and more alert than test scores indicate, causing both caregivers and teachers to perceive them as lazy, stubborn, and unwilling to learn — a faulty perception. If the caregivers are given this information early, frustration for them and for the child may be forestalled.

Burgess (1990) suggests an environmental inventory for preschool children that asks questions about the child's daily life and activities. For example, if a parent answers "no" to the question, "Do you take your child to the grocery store?" the reason could be that the child displays challenging behaviors, for example, temper tantrums. The parent, teacher, and provider can then begin to view the behavior as a communication and shape it appropriately.

Caregivers should also be told about the child's need for consistent structure in the home environment and that the child may require much bodily contact. Ways of providing immediate reinforcement in discipline and setting reasonable goals should also be discussed before behavior becomes a problem. Some children have had abusive or neglectful home situations before they were placed with the present family; counseling may be needed to help the caregivers with symptoms that may occur as a result, such as withdrawal, inappropriate sexual activity, fears, and excessive demand of adults' time and attention (Streissguth et al., 1988).

Children with alcohol-related disorders have some particular health needs: treatment for otitis media, eye problems, eating disorders, and dental needs. They should be seen for regular check-ups by a physician who is aware of the diagnosis.

A service coordinator may be assigned through P.L. 99-457 guidelines. The service coordinator can be the liaison between the family and the school, health personnel, counseling services, and a support group.

Encouraging preschool attendance is important to prepare the children for the school setting ahead. An extra year in a class for the speech and language impaired or in a developmental kindergarten may also be helpful.

The service coordinator may also help to secure respite care for the family. An opportunity to get away from the responsibility of caring for such a child may be crucial to the caregivers' ability to keep doing a good job. This may involve substitute child care, specialized foster care with state reimbursement, or a camp experience for the child.

Interventions for Early School Year

If the child is diagnosed for the first time at school age, the recommendations for infancy are still appropriate with a few exceptions (Table 6–2). Health issues may need treatment rather than preventive care. Referral to specialists may be necessary, the most frequent being orthodontists for dental anomalies, orthopedists and radiologists for skeletal problems, ophthalmologists for vision problems and congenital eye malformations, and cardiologists for heart problems. Therapy for language, articulation, and pragmatics is appropriate, keeping in mind that nontraditional approaches and concrete situations, as discussed in the guidelines, are needed. Children will need more help as language

TABLE 6–2
Interventions for early school years

Provide safe, stable environment

Provide careful, continued monitoring of health issues and existing problems

Provide psychological/educational/adaptive evaluation on regular basis

Provide appropriate educational placement

Provide clear, concrete, and immediate consequences for inappropriate behavior

Encourage respite care

Provide service coordinator as liaison between parents and schools, health providers, and social service agents

---

Source: Adapted from Streissguth et al. (1988, 1990).

tasks become more complex in school, particularly when synthesis of information is required around fourth grade.

Interventions for Adolescents

Maintaining structure and monitoring of the home and school environments become critically important in adolescence in view of sexual behavior (Table 6–3). For caregivers the problem is to permit freedom appropriate to the child's developmental level, while providing enough structure for protection and growth. Streissguth et al. (1988) recommend the Social Skills and Sex Education Guide (Thiel, Nelson, Alrick, & Brodsky, 1977).

Rather than the academic development of the child, a more constructive focus would be to teach vocational, survival, and daily living skills. Adolescents need help with pragmatic language skills involved with managing money, looking after their own health, looking after their appearance and clothes, and making purchases.

For adolescents with FAS who qualify for developmental disabilities services, the transition to services such as sheltered living and workshops is less problematic than for those who do not qualify. For the latter group, adolescence can be particularly difficult; they are aware that they are somehow different and are unable to meet the expectations of others. They may become depressed, and psychological counseling should be an option for them.

Respite care is just as important for the caregivers of adolescents and adults with FAS as it was when their charges were younger. Many

TABLE 6–3
Interventions for adolescents

Provide careful monitoring of social acitivities and structuring of leisure time

Provide education to caretakers and patients regarding sex and birth control

Continue safe, stable environment

Shift educational focus from academic to vocational and living skills

Implement planning for adult residential/vocational training and placement

Provide appropriate mental health intervention if needed

Encourage respite care

Source: Adapted from Streissguth et al. (1988, 1990).

parent support groups work out arrangements so that caregivers may leave their adolescents and adults with FAS with substitute caregivers for periods of time so that they may counteract "burn-out." They should be encouraged to do so (Burgess & Streissguth, 1990).

◧ WHAT SCHOOL DISTRICTS CAN DO

The following are some suggestions for a large-scale effort, most appropriately begun by school districts at an organizational level (Burgess & Streissguth, 1992).

1. **Include questions about prenatal alcohol and drug exposure in the district health screening protocol.** We know little about students' prenatal exposures because we simply do not ask. The questions must be asked in a sensitive, nonjudgmental way, and asking questions should be routine.

2. **Develop a plan for use and distribution of information gathered from health screening.** Districts must consider use of such information very carefully. The purpose is not to stigmatize parents or their children. Responsible planning at the district level can ensure confidentiality and still make this valuable information available to the appropriate professionals.

3. **Provide educational opportunities for district personnel regarding FAS and FAE.** All personnel should have access to appropriate information. Districts can provide inservice opportunities for teachers, paraprofessionals, special service providers (including speech-language pathologists), administrators, and parents.

4. **Develop a referral system for students identified as having possible alcohol or drug related effects.** Once school personnel acquire information about these conditions, they must have guidelines for referring students suspected of having FAS or FAE. FAS is a medical diagnosis and cannot be made by school personnel. Guidelines for referral are provided in Chapter 5. Failure to provide such a referral system may leave school personnel frustrated and possibly unwilling to confront this sensitive issue.

5. **Develop a district-wide plan for meeting the needs of students with known or suspected effects.** School districts must develop a comprehensive plan for serving this

group of students. Such plans are highly specific to the needs and resources of individual communities. Establishing eligibility for services, providing services, and maintaining liaison with families must be considered.

◨ WHAT STATES CAN DO

Service delivery policy begins with the states' interpretation of the laws for education of the handicapped, P.L. 99-457 and P.L. 94-142 (see Chapter 8). One state has created a service delivery system that can serve as a model for others.

Include FAS as Eligible for Intervention Services

Pennsylvania has created an entitlement program for all eligible young children and their families. All eligible children, birth through 2 years of age, are entitled to early intervention services provided by the Pennsylvania Department of Public Welfare. Eligible children include children who are experiencing developmental delays or have a physical or mental condition that has a high probability of resulting in a developmental delay, including FAS (Antoniadis & Daulton, 1992).

Establish a Tracking System for FAS Children Who Do Not Receive Intervention

Pennsylvania also mandates interagency collaboration to identify, screen, and track children who are at risk from birth through 5 years of age. Children eligible for tracking and monitoring include "children born to chemically dependent mothers." This includes children with FAS. However, to become eligible for full entitlement, they must be developmentally delayed. Eligibility is based on developmental needs of children, assessed in terms of the child's and family's strengths and those things required to achieve optimal functioning. The at-risk screening and tracking system creates a community-based service system for the delivery of identification, monitoring, and referral services. The necessity to identify and monitor children and families who are not immediately eligible for services provides a vehicle to consistently reevaluate progress and assist in obtaining status changes. Interagency coordination of data collection activities strengthens the knowledge base regarding at-risk children as well as those eligible for services (Antoniadis & Daulton, 1992).

▪️🔲 A CAUTION AGAINST STEREOTYPING

At the beginning of the section on age-specific phenotypes, the caution was given that individuals with FAS or FAE will not fit the phenotype. The individuals in the studies cited were born before the general recognition of FAS, and many were not diagnosed until childhood or adolescence. *We do not know the potential for children diagnosed at birth and raised in nurturant homes with appropriate programming.* We would do a great disservice to "pigeon-hole" all affected children with this label and lower our expectations to fit the phenotypes described earlier. Even as we guard against stereotyping, we must add to our knowledge of the limitations that prenatal alcohol abuse places on a child. Streissguth et al. (1988) likewise remind of us our challenge.

> Recognition of these limitations can help the family plan effectively for future needs as well as provide appropriate remedial experiences to enhance the level of adaptive functioning.... The role of the home and school environment becomes critical, (particularly for the most functional patients) in determining whether these patients will become productive happy members of society, or whether they will become isolated, lonely transients, at risk for exploitation, victimization, and feelings of inadequacy. (p. 36)

▪️🔲 SUMMARY

In this chapter we have discussed general guidelines for intervention with children and adolescents with alcohol-related disorders. Interventions are recommended for service providers and teachers. Recommendations for school districts and for state policies have also been provided. To date, interventions for children with alcohol-related disorders are not based on solid evaluation methodologies. In later chapters, methodologies for empirical research with children exposed to prenatal drugs will be discussed, as will methodologies for evaluation of intervention.

Prevention of Prenatal Substance Abuse

A s has been emphasized in previous chapters, women do not begin to drink or use drugs when they are pregnant, rather they become pregnant while they are drinking or using drugs. If we are to prevent the effects of prenatal exposure to drugs and alcohol, women must either not expose their fetus, knowingly or unknowingly, because they do not abuse drugs or, with the knowledge that they are pregnant, must limit or abstain from substance use for the remainder of the pregnancy. Data published in the medical literature tell us that if we can identify the pregnant drug- or alcohol-using woman early in pregnancy, provide obstetric care, get her into treatment, and bring her to abstinence by the second or third trimester, we can prevent many of the harmful effects of the drug or alcohol on the child. The next step is to begin developing programs that will move us into the arena of prevention, programs that will reach men and women of child-bearing age, programs that will eliminate all chances of drug use by pregnant women (Chasnoff, 1991).

There is good news in recent evidence that the number of women who consume alcohol during pregnancy is declining. However, it also appears that the rates of alcohol consumption among high-risk populations (pregnant smokers, unmarried women, women under the age of 25, and women with the least amount of education) remain virtually unchanged (Serdula, Williamson, Kendrick, Anda, & Byers, 1991). This points to a need to target prevention and education efforts to reach high-risk populations and to identify women at high risk (Gordis, 1992).

In this chapter, we will focus on the substance-using mother instead of her child. The prevention efforts described here are feasible for school-based personnel. Traditionally, school personnel are most often involved with so-called *primary* prevention efforts — those that provide education about the dangers of substance abuse in pregnancy. As we become more involved with families, we have opportunities for *secondary* prevention efforts as well — identification of the substance abuser and those at high risk. Research is now available about the relative effectiveness of these efforts. *Tertiary* prevention, in this discussion, means treatment for alcoholism or substance abuse disorders for the woman; again, not every approach is effective, particularly for women. Teachers and service providers also refer women to treatment. The goal of treatment is abstinence, or at least abstinence while pregnant. Voluntary treatment modalities, mandatory treatment, and prosecution will be discussed to provide an overview of treatment facilities and barriers to treatment for women.

A great deal of progress has been made in the United States in approaches to preventing and treating alcoholism and other drug addictions among women. Prior to the 1970s there were virtually no treatment options for women with alcoholism and other drug addictions. Women rarely came into treatment; when they did, the treatment they received was based on the male experience of alcoholism with no adjustments for the fact that a woman's life experience and physiology are different from a man's.

The 1970s were a time of dramatic change for women in need of treatment for alcoholism and other drug addictions. The National Institute on Alcohol Abuse and Alcoholism (NIAA) funded the first wave of women's treatment programs across the nation. Later, in 1984, the women's set-aside of the Alcohol, Drug Abuse and Mental-Health Services (ADMS) block grant required that states spend 5% of their block grant award on new prevention and treatment efforts designed for women. The set-aside requirement was raised in 1988 to 10%.

Only a few prevention and treatment efforts have focused specifically on pregnant alcoholic and other drug-dependent pregnant women. Service providers are concerned about potential liability problems associated with treating pregnant, addicted women. There is also a great need for additional training of treatment providers about how to proceed with safe detoxification and treatment. To date, much of the reaction to treating pregnant alcoholic and other drug-dependent women has been guided by fear, lack of knowledge, and lack of experience. The sad irony is that pregnancy offers an opportunity to intervene and provide treatment, yet it is at this very time that the least amount of treatment is available (NCADD, 1990).

The Anti-Drug Abuse Act of 1988 included a provision to establish prevention, education, intervention, and treatment demonstration projects administered through the Office for Substance Abuse Prevention for pregnant and postpartum alcoholic and other drug-dependent women. This program has stimulated the development of some of the first programs in the nation to address the needs of pregnant women (NCADD, 1990).

■ CONCEPTUAL FRAMEWORK

Before we look at specific prevention efforts and their relative effectiveness, it is helpful to discuss how people make decisions that affect their health and well-being. Those decisions are based on social learning theory, in which the pioneers were Fishbein and Ajzen (1975). Very simply put, they believed that people decide on a health action according to the norm in one's culture, that is, do other people whom one values think something is important? For example, if one's group of friends takes their children for innoculations, then the new mother in that group will probably do likewise. If, on the other hand, getting an innoculation is a rare thing in one's neighborhood, the forces that sway a new mother to take her child for a shot must be strong enough to overcome the normative influence. It is easy to see alcohol and drug use in that light. A woman who lives in an environment where substances are used, even during pregnancy, will not be likely to view that behavior as out of the ordinary. The influence of the peer group is strong in substance behavior and not easily overcome. Our focus is on a woman's health-related behavior and how she decides to take a particular action or not. The example used throughout this section is the decision to seek recovery treatment for an alcohol or drug abuse problem. Let us assume that a woman has heard the media campaigns — that drinking or drug use while pregnant may cause birth defects. What factors go into her decision to change her behavior? Two behaviors are possible: to continue as she has or to change her drug use behavior. The conceptual framework for this discussion includes the Health Belief Model (HBM) and the concept of self-efficacy.

Health Belief Model

For more than three decades, the Health Belief Model has been one of the most influential and widely used psychosocial approaches to explaining health-related behavior (Rosenstock, 1990). People will most likely follow a health recommendation if they have an incentive and if they hold four separate beliefs:

1. That they are vulnerable — perceived susceptibility.
2. That the disease can have a serious impact on their lives — perceived severity. The combination of susceptibility and severity is labeled as *perceived threat.*
3. That following the recommendation will reduce the severity —perceived benefits.
4. That the benefits outweigh the barriers — perceived barriers.

The health belief model can be seen as an equation:

$$Behavior = [Susceptibility \times Severity] \times [Benefits - Barriers]$$

Perceived Susceptibility

The dimension of perceived susceptibility refers to one's perception of risk. Does a woman believe that she or her fetus could be harmed by this substance? If she believes that she can escape this harm, her perceived susceptibility may be very low. That low perception may be reinforced because other women in her environment took the same substance while pregnant with no apparent harm to the baby.

Perceived Severity

Perceived severity refers to her perception of just how serious the consequences would be. Some women take cocaine to induce labor so that they will have a smaller and easier-to-deliver baby. That consequence is not perceived to be as severe as a lifelong disability.

Perceived Benefits

Perceived threat does not define the specific course of action to be taken. This depends on beliefs regarding the effectiveness of the various available actions in reducing the threat, or the perceived benefits of taking an action. Thus an individual would not be expected to accept any recommended action unless that action was perceived as feasible and efficacious (Rosenstock, 1990).

Perceived Barriers

Perceived barriers may act as impediments to undertaking the recommended behavior. A kind of unconscious, cost-benefit analysis is thought to occur wherein the individual weighs an action's effectiveness against perceptions that it may be expensive, dangerous, unpleasant, inconvenient, time-consuming, and so forth. Thus, "the combined levels of susceptibility and severity provided the energy or force to act and the perception of benefits (less barriers) provided a preferred path of action" (Rosenstock, 1974, p. 332).

Self-Efficacy

Another dimension must be added to the HBM. For behavior change to succeed, people must feel threatened by their current behavioral patterns (perceived susceptibility and severity) and believe that change of a specific kind will be beneficial and result in a valued outcome at acceptable cost, but they must also feel themselves competent (self-efficacious) to implement that change (Rosenstock, 1990). Self-efficacy is defined as "the conviction that one can successfully execute the behavior required to produce the outcomes" (Bandura, 1977, p. 79). Self-efficacy is specific to a situation and is not the same as general self-confidence. A person with high self-efficacy can have one set-back or relapse but continue to try for sobriety. A person with low self-efficacy may give up after one relapse. Self-efficacy can determine whether a woman thinks she can get rid of an addiction. For example, for a woman to quit drinking during pregnancy, she must not only believe that cessation will benefit the health of her baby but also that she is capable of quitting.

Changing Self-Efficacy

Pregnancy has been called a window of opportunity for getting a woman into treatment. This suggests that pregnancy can indeed be a time when women may be motivated to tackle their addiction (Chavkin, 1991). How can one's self-efficacy, especially about giving up alcohol or a drug, be boosted? External forces can begin to change self-efficacy, but it must be internalized to make it stick. For example, a woman may be given information on the dangers of substance abuse in pregnancy and urged by those close to her to quit her use, but until she is motivated herself, she is unlikely to change her self-efficacy. Ways to change self-efficacy are:

1. *Obtain information.* Certainly information is important for behavior change. Too often it is seen as all that is necessary. In the past, prevention programs were almost completely informational. Most were based on the premise that sufficient knowledge about alcohol and other drugs would preclude their use (Goodstadt, 1978). Efforts to change cognitions about health matters have often involved attempts to arouse fear through threatening messages (Rosenstock, 1990). Messages from the media play on those fears. If people become too fearful, however, this tactic can backfire. It is well known that a pamphlet with the words "Drugs" or "Alcohol" on the front will not be picked up by pregnant women as often as one with words such as "Baby care," or "How to have a healthy baby." Evaluation of information programs is discussed later in this chapter.

2. *Remove the emotional overlay.* Seeking treatment requires admitting that there is a problem with substance use. A woman and her family may be protecting her and themselves from having to acknowledge that she needs help and be caught in denial. Others in the family may actively oppose treatment of any kind. Women who are identified as the wife and mother in the family often think that they have failed morally (Roth, 1991).

3. *Model the behavior.* Teachers and service providers know that this is a vital step in the process of changing behavior. In this context, modeling behavior can mean that someone else in the woman's social environment has changed her substance behavior. It could also mean that a woman chooses to remain in a social group that supports her efforts because abstinence is the normative behavior of the group.

4. *Have a success.* Some period of sobriety should be looked at as a success, even if it does not last and relapse occurs. Even taking a step toward seeking treatment, such as making a phone call, should be pointed out as a success. "You took the first step. You called. Now you have to go to the meeting."

Research on Prevention Approaches

Not all prevention approaches are effective. In this section, research findings on some of the most common primary and secondary prevention efforts will be explored.

Information

Evaluations of programs that focus on providing factual information as their primary strategy indicate that increased knowledge alone has virtually no effect on subsequent abuse (Botvin, 1983). Strategies that have their roots in social learning theory hold more promise (Bandura, 1977).

Minor and Van Dort (1982) studied the effect of media information about FAS and the effect of discussing drinking while pregnant with a doctor or nurse on a sample of women who had just given birth in Los Angeles County. Although 96% of the sample had heard or read that, if a pregnant woman drinks alcohol, it can harm her unborn child, only 55% stated that they had heard or read about FAS. Of those who had heard about FAS, they were in agreement with current knowledge about FAS with the exception that 50% thought that FAS could be cured. These results suggest that, on the one hand, women's risky drinking practices during pregnancy were relatively independent of exposure to or knowledge about the teratogenic effects of alcohol. On the other hand, not discussing drinking alcohol during pregnancy with a doctor or nurse increased the likelihood of women's risky drinking practices during pregnancy.

Information Based on Fear

A purely informational or fear-based approach is largely ineffective in altering behavior, although it may increase knowledge. The literature on the use of drugs and alcohol indicates only a fairly modest relationship among changes in knowledge, attitudes, and behavior. When these programs led to behavior change, the changes were often small and usually involved delaying the onset of a behavior rather than preventing it altogether (Gomby & Larson, 1992; Rundall & Bruvold, 1988).

School Curriculum

The literature indicates that a fact-based curriculum alone is not sufficient to change student behavior. Early efforts to prevent risky health behaviors — smoking, alcohol or drug abuse — employed heavily information-based or fear-laden messages. Gradually, research discredited these curricula because they tended to influence student knowledge but not behavior (Forman & Linney, 1988; Goodstadt, 1978). Today, the most up-to-date programs involve curricula that are based on social learning theories. Such curricula provide students with information as well as training in social skills to resist pressures from peers, family, or the media; with skills to make thoughtful decisions about health behaviors; and with opportunities to role-play and practice their skills (Gomby & Larson, 1992).

Warning Labels

Congress passed legislation requiring health warnings to be printed on all bottles and cans of alcohol sold in the United States in 1989. Although women are increasingly aware of the labels, it has not had much effect on their drinking habits. Labels, even combined with warnings from physicians, are not enough (Hankin & Firestone, 1992). Other factors have been shown to play a greater role in the decision to drink than knowledge of the warning label, including history of heavy drinking, older age, and personal attitudes.

Posters

A growing number of communities now require FAS warning posters at points of purchase for alcoholic beverages. This vehicle has proved to be a potent means, in conjunction with broader educational campaigns, of raising public awareness about the risks to the fetus of drinking during pregnancy. The National Council on Alcoholism's New York affiliate mounted a successful legislative campaign to post warning signs in liquor stores, bars, and restaurants in 1983 (NCADD, 1983). Their presence has had a substantial educational effect. A Gallup poll found that after the first year in which the signs were in place, New Yorkers' awareness of the dangers to the fetus of drinking during pregnancy rose from 56% to 68%.

Screening for High-Risk Women

Another method is to give screening questionnaires for alcohol and drug problems to women in programs such as the WIC (Women Infants and Children). WIC is a supplementary food program for pregnant, postpartum, and breast-feeding women and for infants and children whose health is threatened by both low income and nutritional need. The University of Nebraska Medical Center's WIC office found 5.5% of 947 women screened to be at high risk for alcohol abuse and actively involved with alcohol during the pregnancy. More than 21% were found to be at moderate risk. These women were not actively drinking but were involved with alcohol before the pregnancy and had family members and friends who drank. Women identified at high risk were urged to get counseling on site or were referred to outside agencies like Alcoholics Anonymous (*University of Nebraska Medical Center News*, 1988). The screener, *Do You Know the Facts* (Alcohol and Drug Abuse Council of Nebraska, 1988), is now used at all WIC programs in Nebraska as a means of referring women for drug and alcohol counseling in their own communities.

Public Education Campaigns

Many public education campaigns have been sponsored by both governmental and private agencies. These campaigns have been effective in increasing general public knowledge, but have not affected the number of heavy drinkers. The failure to change behavior among those at highest risk may be linked to the message content (fear and punishment) and the inability of public campaigns to treat addiction (Little, Young, Streissguth, & Uhl, 1984).

Prenatal Care

Randall (1991) reported that an "intensive" prenatal care program (seeing the same obstetrician every 2 weeks from the point of enrollment in the program until delivery) can influence a woman's ability to become drug free, carry her infant to term, and keep her child after it is born far more than had been previously recognized. Although the effect of the program on women's behavior was short-term, and many of the women went back to their drug habit, the program was successful in getting babies into the world who were clean at the time of birth and did not have to spend months in the neonatal intensive care unit.

Counseling

Supportive counseling has been demonstrated to be effective in reducing consumption among women at risk and in improving pregnancy outcome (Morse, Weiner, & Garrido, 1989). In another study (Rosett, Weiner, & Edelin, 1983) of pregnant problem drinkers who participated in at least three counseling sessions, 67% reduced alcohol consumption before the third trimester.

■ PREVENTION CLASSIFICATIONS

With the framework and research conclusions just discussed in mind, prevention classifications will be considered. Guidelines will be given on how teachers and service providers can participate. Traditionally, prevention programs have been classified as primary, secondary, and tertiary, depending on where on the continuum of use of alcohol and other drugs the intervention takes place.

Primary Prevention

Because disorders caused by prenatal substance abuse are preventable, the implications for primary prevention are clear. Anything that can be done to prevent or decrease substance use during pregnancy should decrease the prevalence of the disorders.

The goal of primary, or early, prevention is to defer or preclude initiation of involvement with alcohol and other drugs. Examples of targeted individuals may be youth near the age of onset of risk, with no prior involvement with alcohol or other drugs, or youth who have just begun use but do not show a pattern of abuse. In the development of such efforts, the concept of personal responsibility for the initial decision to use or refrain from use of substances should be emphasized (American Medical Association, 1991).

Primary Prevention Activities for Teachers and Service Providers

Some of the activities described next can only be done in the school setting. There is no reason to limit oneself to those activities, however. Individuals can be active in community and legislative efforts as well.

Volunteer to talk with junior high and high school classes. Educational programs about alcohol and other drugs attempt to increase students' knowledge about the legal, pharmacological, and medical consequences of abusing these substances. Some topics to include are:

1. Parenting begins at conception, not at birth;
2. Dangers of alcohol and drugs while pregnant;
3. Dangers of breast feeding while using alcohol and drugs;
4. Dangers of passive cocaine and marijuana smoke.

Take part in public education and school health activities. Reaching the general public, especially women of childbearing age, with information about alcohol-related birth defects is a major thrust of most FAS/FAE prevention programs such as Fetal Alcohol Prevention Week, sponsored by the National Council on Alcoholism and Drug Dependence. Such public education campaigns should not be limited to women of childbearing age; informed mothers, friends, and spouses may also serve as informal educators. Print materials, community education programs, and mass media are complementary and reinforcing modes of communication that reach a broad cross-section of the community (Ronan,

1985). Literature can be distributed at appropriate places outside the school where pregnant women may see it. Posters and pamphlets are the most common print materials developed and distributed by FAS/FAE prevention programs. Some excellent locations for placing such materials are doctors' offices, pharmacies, laboratories where pregnancy tests and premarital and pregnancy blood tests are taken, marriage license bureaus, social service agencies, church bulletins, maternity clothing stores, children's clothing stores, shopping mall displays, state liquor stores, supermarkets, family planning services, health clubs, WIC nutrition programs, laundromats, prepared childbirth classes, YWCAs, other women's clubs, beauty shops, and many other places frequented by women (Yancosek, 1982).

Presentations that provide more detailed information through the use of speakers and audiovisual materials are effective mechanisms for increasing awareness. Such programs can be offered to the membership of existing organizations, clubs, and groups such as childbirth education classes, LeLeche, PTAs, and YWCAs. All presentations should emphasize the positive aspects of healthy pregnancies rather than the negative aspects of birth defects. Some schools and communities have established a speaker's bureau composed of experts on various aspects of drug and alcohol abuse (Ronan, 1985).

Newspapers, radio, television, and magazines are also useful channels for communicating information about alcohol-related birth defects. A sample spot announcement is shown in Figure 7–1.

Take part in developing school curriculum materials that carry a message on alcohol and drugs. To ensure that information on alcohol-related birth defects reaches teenagers before alcohol becomes a problem, it should be incorporated at all levels of education under the heading of preventing developmental disabilities. The Nebraska alcohol-and-drug school curriculum, (Beardsley, Gillespie, & Williams, 1985) includes junior and senior high school units on alcohol, drugs, and pregnancy. Most states, however, do not include such information in the elementary school curriculum. Curriculum materials should be based on social learning theory instead of fact-based for best results.

Take part in inservice presentations about alcohol and drugs. Once training and inservices have been provided, a prevention program should continue to provide ongoing services as an information and referral source. Periodic training is, of course, necessary to reach newly identified providers (Ronan, 1985).

Work for legislation for increased labeling on bottles containing alcohol and display of posters to warn pregnant women of the dangers of their use. A number of communities have found that the very activity of launching a

30-SECONDS

SAY NO. AND SAY YES TO YOUR LIFE.

THE NATIONAL COUNCIL ON ALCOHOLISM WANTS TO SAVE LIVES BY TEACHING KIDS TO SAY NO TO ALCOHOL AND OTHER DRUGS.

THERE'S ANOTHER ALCOHOL TRAGEDY THAT WOMEN HAVE THE POWER TO PREVENT. FETAL ALCOHOL SYNDROME — FAS. FAS IS THE THIRD LEADING CAUSE OF BIRTH DEFECTS WITH ACCOMPANYING MENTAL RETARDATION. IT'S THE ONLY ONE OF THE TOP THREE THAT'S COMPLETELY PREVENTABLE.

SO PLEASE, IF YOU'RE PLANNING FOR MOTHERHOOD, SAY NO TO ALCOHOL AND OTHER DRUGS. AND SAY YES TO YOUR BABY'S LIFE.

20-SECONDS

PREGNANT? . . . THEN, THINK ABOUT THIS: EVERY TIME YOU TAKE A DRINK, SO DOES YOUR BABY . . . AND ALCOHOL CAN CAUSE IRREVERSIBLE BIRTH DEFECTS . . . (Your agency's name) AND (call letters of station) WANT TO HELP YOU ENJOY A HEALTHY BABY . . . CALL _____ .

10-SECONDS

IF YOU ARE PREGNANT, AVOID ALCOHOL. ALCOHOL CAN BE HAZARDOUS TO YOUR UNBORN BABY'S HEALTH. FOR MORE INFORMATION ON FETAL ALCOHOL SYNDROME, CALL _____ .

10-SECONDS

THIS IS FETAL ALCOHOL SYNDROME AWARENESS WEEK. (Station) AND (Agency) REMIND YOU: ALCOHOL IS A DRUG AND NOT FOR PREGNANT WOMEN.

Figure 7-1
Sample FAS public service radio announcements. These sample PSAs were provided by the NCA-Alabama Division, the Illinois Department of Alcoholism and Drug Abuse, and the National Council on Alcoholism.

warning poster initiative is in itself an important opportunity for raising awareness as well as a chance to bring together disparate constituency groups to support an alcohol-related public health initiative. Furthermore, such efforts ultimately strengthen national and state public policy initiatives relating to health warning labeling of product containers and advertising.

Secondary Prevention

The goal of this second level of prevention is to identify persons in the early stages of problem behaviors associated with alcohol and other drugs and to avert the ensuing negative consequences by inducing them to cease their use through counseling or other treatment. This requires attention to the early behavioral and physical signs that were pointed out in Chapter 2. Programs at this level should incorporate components for identifying individuals who need medical treatment or counseling and for making appropriate referrals to community resources (Botvin, 1983).

Secondary Prevention Activities for Teachers and Service Providers

These activities are most likely to be appropriate for professionals involved in early intervention and especially for those who are home visitors.

Work to get a mother who has one affected child into treatment to prevent another affected child. When we see an infant with FAS, it is a signal of a mother at risk, of a child with special needs, and of a high-risk environment.

- ◼️ Work to get any woman who is pregnant and using drugs or alcohol into prenatal care.
- ◼️ Be very emphatic about the mother not breast feeding while she is using drugs or alcohol.
- ◼️ Be vigilant for cocaine or marijuana smoke in the home.
- ◼️ Refer to treatment or counseling. Tell the woman that cutting down will help. At the very least she can be urged to call one of the Helpline numbers listed in Appendix B.

Tertiary Prevention

The outcome of the third level of prevention is to end compulsive use of alcohol or other drugs or to ameliorate its negative effects through treatment and rehabilitation of the mother (American Medical Association, 1991). Women tend to enter treatment later in their disease process than men do. If their problem is alcohol, women tend to be misdiagnosed by physicians and are often given other medications for their symptoms of depression. According to Little and Wendt (1991), the less developed the drinking problem, the greater the treatment success rate and the better the pregnancy outcome. Women in the later stages of alcoholism are at a very high risk and have the most severely affected children. While an ideal outcome would be immediate and permanent abstinence, some women cannot immediately cease all use. Thus, for some users the only realistic goal may be to reduce the use of the drugs for the duration of the pregnancy.

Teachers and service providers are not drug counselors nor should they try to provide recovery treatment. Our tertiary prevention efforts concern referral for treatment. Therefore, no guidelines for school personnel are given. Instead, an overview of services and research available on their effectiveness and important barriers to women for obtaining treatment are provided.

Finally, if a woman will not voluntarily curtail her drug and alcohol use while pregnant, should mandatory treatment be an option? Should a woman who continues her drug or alcohol use be punished for it after she has a child affected by that use?

Many experts believe that the most effective treatment model for pregnant, drug-dependent women is the comprehensive model program. The following services should be included in a model program: (1) staff that is trained and sensitive to pregnant addicts' issues; (2) provision of adequate physical, interpersonal, and social supports; (3) family involvement in therapy and child care; (4) obstetric, pediatric, and medical care for women and infants; and (5) educational and vocational assistance (Finnegan, 1979). Comprehensive programs, such as the NAPARE program described in Chapter 4, are very rare.

Treatment Modalities

Drug treatment services are offered through a variety of modalities, relying on either a residential or outpatient approach. Within these categories, there is substantial variation. In residential programs, there are both long-term therapeutic communities and short-term drug dependency hospitals or treatment centers. Within outpatient programs there are programs that involve frequent and intensive counselling and others that consist of one or two hourly sessions per week. The following is a general description of four major treatment modalities (Kumpfer, 1991).

- *Residential Therapeutic Communities.* This type of program targets the most heavily impaired, polydrug users. It removes drug users from their environment and immerses them in a structured intensive program. These programs often revolve around a set of norms and a system of rewards and punishment. The client is expected to comply with this system and often to participate in the housework and other tasks of communal living. These programs typically do not allow children of clients to live in the residence and thus require some other custody arrangement for any children. The length of stay in such a program can vary, but it most often is for several months or even a year.

- *Residential Drug Treatment Centers.* This is the most widely used treatment modality, probably because it typically is covered by private insurance policies. Like therapeutic communities, these centers also target highly impaired drug and/or alcohol users. They also provide a residential, highly structured program, but for a shorter period of 14–28 days. Like therapeutic communities, these programs usually do not allow children to live at the center. Unlike therapeutic communities, these drug treatment centers do not typically require the client to participate in the chores of communal living.

- *Outpatient-Intensive.* Some residential programs have developed daily outpatient programs for clients who require intensive therapy but cannot live at the center. This type of program can be an attractive alternative for clients with children, but the programs must be located near where the client lives, or be easily accessible by public transportation.

- *Outpatient.* This category has the most diversity of programs. Typically, outpatient programs, which target less impaired drug users, are less expensive than residential and intensive outpatient services. These programs are offered by a vast array of providers, including drop-in centers, community mental health programs, self-help groups, clergy, and private counselors. Few, however, provide ancillary services geared toward children, such as child care, parent education, and prenatal and perinatal health care.

All of these residential and outpatient programs rely on different therapeutic approaches, with one of the most common being the 12–step program used in Alcoholics Anonymous (AA), in which patients follow the 12 steps of AA to grow mentally, emotionally, and spiritually. This approach stresses individual responsibility and recovery, rather than family therapy.

Cocaine Recovery and 12-Step Programs

The treatment of cocaine abusers is a newly emerging discipline. Many of the strategies being developed for this purpose have been adapted from the drug and alcoholism treatment systems. These include use of established programs that are only minimally modified for cocaine abusers, such as the 28-day inpatient hospital, therapeutic community, and 12-step programs (Rawson, Obert, McCann, Castro, & Ling, 1991).

A detailed discussion of the 12-step program of Alcoholics Anonymous (AA) is beyond the scope of this book. As cocaine abusers have sought assistance for their problem, many have used the support and guidance provided by the 12-step programs. In fact, the movement of cocaine abusers into AA meetings became so overwhelming that a separate organization, Cocaine Anonymous (CA), was established as a 12-step support system for cocaine abusers. Cocaine Anonymous has spread rapidly (Rawson et al., 1991).

There has been little research to evaluate the usefulness of AA or CA for cocaine abusers. Clearly, those who do attend and become cocaine abstinent are tremendously loyal to the 12-step program. Much popular press coverage has focused on the positive impact that AA and CA have provided for recovering cocaine abusers. Many recovering cocaine users credit AA and CA as being the foundation for their recovery progress. They have contributed to the popular assumption that the only proper way to achieve and maintain cocaine abstinence is through involvement with 12-step programs (Rawson et al., 1991).

Articles have been written about the limitations of 12-step programs, and case studies have described damage from AA/CA involvement. These programs are not professionally run treatment organizations that can tailor the materials for specific individual needs. Some people are not helped by involvement in 12-step programs. Many more do not attend enough meetings to be able to determine if the meetings might be of benefit. However, on balance, the best current recommendation is to encourage cocaine abusers to sample a number of AA and/or CA meetings. If they find they do receive some benefit from their involvement, continued attendance should be reinforced and encouraged. If they do not find participation useful, they should be provided other types of treatment assistance without penalty for noninvolvement in 12-step programs (Rawson et al., 1991). Twelve-step programs require adequate cognitive abilities and literacy.

Research on Treatment Effectiveness

Data have repeatedly indicated that concern for children often motivates addicted women to seek drug treatment and that lack of services for children precludes women's ongoing participation (Chavkin, 1991).

Unfortunately, relatively little is known from scientific research about the effectiveness of different modalities of treatment for drug abuse. Furthermore, what is known has been developed primarily from studies involving men. We do know that despite the uncertainty about treatment effectiveness, the demand for treatment is much greater than the supply. The vast majority of programs now treat both drug and alcohol problems (Kumpfer, 1991).

The least amount of research exists about the effects of short-term, inpatient drug treatment centers, but this category of program usually absorbs the most revenues. The Institute of Medicine (IOM) (1990) found that "there are no relevant experimental or quasi-experimental studies" of this type of treatment modality, and "the extent of reasonable certain knowledge" is limited to knowing that clients treated for alcohol problems have better outcomes than those treated for drug problems. Most of the studies available have reported treatment outcomes in terms of drug use, criminality, and employability. They did not consider proper childrearing in their outcome analysis. The question arises as to whether the results of these studies are applicable to women, let alone pregnant women and children.

Barriers to Women

Only a small percentage of addicted women ever enter a substance-abuse treatment program. The IOM Committee (1990) estimated that there are approximately 105,000 pregnant women each year who need drug treatment. Only 30,000 of these women receive any form of treatment, and very few of those who do are in programs with a primary focus on special services for pregnant women.

This unmet demand extends throughout the country. In 1985, Kumpfer and Holman found in Utah that only about 7.3% of all women abusing drugs and alcohol were receiving treatment. Women in urban areas were much more likely to receive treatment (17.8%) than women in rural, isolated areas (2.2%). Only 13.5% of the clients in treatment facilities were women (down from 28% in 1978). Furst, Beckman, Nakamura, and Weiss (1981) reported for California that there were four times more men than women in publicly funded treatment, and two-

and-a-half times more men than women in all treatment programs, public or private.

Four primary obstacles to treatment may explain why such a low percentage of women receive treatment (Kumpfer, 1991):

1. *Lack of women's treatment facilities and programs.* Two thirds of major hospitals in 15 cities included in a 1989 survey commissioned by the House Select Committee on Children, Youth and Families reported they had no place to refer drug-dependent women for treatment (Miller, 1989). The major factors contributing to this deficit are inadequate public funding for drug treatment for women and the exclusion of pregnant women from most existing treatment programs.

2. *Exclusion of pregnant women and women with children.* Even treatment programs that accept women often refuse to admit women who are pregnant. Treatment programs cite numerous legal and medical concerns as justification for excluding pregnant women: concerns about detoxification during pregnancy, lack of prenatal care, lack of facilities for the infant when born if the woman is in a long-term residential program, and their inability to become a licensed child care facility or nursery. Few drug treatment services can accommodate women with children either through outpatient treatment with child care or in a residential program for mothers with their children (Kumpfer, 1991).

Formidable barriers discourage drug and alcohol treatment programs from meeting the housing, child care, and other social needs of drug-abusing mothers. Thus, women with children, particularly older children, must often choose between continuing custody and care for their children and drug treatment (Kumpfer, 1991).

3. *Lack of treatment programs sensitive to women's needs.* Additional barriers to treatment include program accessibility, quality, safety, and attractiveness to women. Treatment programs have targeted men. The realities of addicted women are that they are often (1) poor, unemployed, and lacking in employable job skills; (2) single, divorced, or separated, and often isolated from a social support system; and (3) mothers of children who need their care and attention. For treatment programs to be attractive and responsive to these women, they must recognize their needs and provide the support required to meet those needs (Kumpfer, 1991).

Women may even need a different kind of therapy. Drug-using women, on average, have poorer self-esteem than drug-using men and suffer greater anxiety, depression, and detachment. As a result, reliance on confrontational therapy techniques may worsen such problems rather than help reduce them (Institute of Medicine, 1990).

Finally, improving parenting is an important need for many drug-abusing mothers. It has been suggested that classic therapeutic methodologies have to be modified to meet the needs of this special population and that parenting issues should be a primary focus. Some research does exist concerning the effectiveness of programs for this population. Kumpfer (1985) reported that a comprehensive family skills training program in Salt Lake City, Utah, the Strengthening Families Program, was successful in improving parenting skills of drug-abusing parents and in decreasing behavioral and emotional problems in 6- to 12-year-old children of drug abusers. The NIDA-funded program included 14 weeks of parent training and extensive work with the children alone and the family as a whole. This program has been replicated successfully with black, addicted mothers in Alabama and is being implemented with federal funding from the Office for Substance Abuse Prevention (OSAP) in Detroit, Utah, and Hawaii, where culturally sensitive versions are being developed with local and national consultants (Kumpfer, 1991).

4. *Fear and isolation in women.* A woman who drinks too much or uses drugs is looked down on more than a man who engages in the same behavior. As the stigma, rejection, and blame increase, drug-abusing women's feelings of guilt and shame increase. This leads to lowered self-esteem, increased depression, immobilization, and isolation. As societal stigma increases, willingness to enter treatment decreases (Kumpfer, 1991).

Mandatory Treatment

Because of the crack epidemic and the high level of drug use in young women, there have been attempts to impose criminal sanctions on pregnant women who use drugs or alcohol. There are no research data to substantiate the effectiveness of compulsory treatment in general. Neither outcomes nor comparison groups have been clearly specified. We lack a firm database from which to judge efficacy. However, efficacy is only one measure to be considered when formulating policy; protection of constitutional rights and furtherance of public health and other social goals are critical yardsticks as well. Establishing a policy to compel pregnant women into treatment may exacerbate current social inequities affecting women in general and poor minority women in particular. Furthermore, the evaluative efforts of compulsory treatment have dealt almost exclusively with male subjects. In the United States, mandatory treatment of chemical dependency comprises three general groupings or models (Chavkin, 1991).

1. *Mandatory treatment in the law enforcement context.* This refers to providing treatment as an alternative to trial or incarceration for those arrested or convicted of crimes and found to be drug users. Failure to remain in treatment renders the user liable to criminal prosecution and penalty. Although few data are available, it seems that female addicts who entered drug treatment under legal pressure indicated that they were less likely to remain in treatment than women who entered voluntarily (Chavkin, 1991).

2. *Civil commitment.* This refers to persons diagnosed as addicted and considered incapable of self-care or a potential threat to the public's safety because of their addiction, but who have not been accused or convicted of any crime. These programs have traditionally used settings that were more like prisons than treatment facilities, particularly with the unavailability of treatment facilities. This scarcity has been magnified for pregnant women who have been categorically excluded from most drug treatment programs. Women may be put in jails or prisons where drugs are readily available, but where prenatal care is not.

3. *Treatment mandated as a precondition for obtaining a privilege.* Chemically dependent parents deemed neglectful or abusive are often mandated to receive treatment as a precondition for maintaining or regaining custody of their children. The limited literature on the efficacy of this approach suggests that parents mandated to treatment fare about the same as those who participate voluntarily (Chavkin, 1991).

Both the American College of Obstetrics and Gynecology and the American Medical Association have adopted positions opposing court-ordered medical treatment or penalty in response to behavior by a pregnant woman deemed to jeopardize fetal welfare. Moreover, penalizing approaches that underscore guilt and shame may be counterproductive and deter women from use of such services. In short, mandatory treatment does not seem to achieve the goal of safeguarding the fetus from exposure to drugs or alcohol (Chavkin, 1991).

To be effective, psychological treatment requires the active participation of the patient. As discussed in the section on self-efficacy, although external consequences may motivate the addict to seek treatment, the motivation must be internalized. In the case of mandatory treatment, it is imposed. Resistance to treatment can be manifested in passive resistance and active sabotage (Chavkin, 1991).

Might the purpose of mandatory treatment of a pregnant woman be to improve her level of parental functioning? Providing her with treatment and support while she raises her child might achieve that goal, whereas mandating treatment during pregnancy and discharging her postpartum, especially with the relapse-provoking stresses of new motherhood, seems unlikely to attain it. Such an approach also implicitly negates the role of the father. It not only assumes parental responsibility to be solely maternal, but also ignores the potential male contribution to female drug use. Many women report initiation into drug use by male sex partners, as well as sabotage of their efforts to abstain from drugs by their drug-using partners. If the goal of mandatory treatment during pregnancy is to improve parental functioning, then its achievement requires including fathers and extending treatment beyond birth (Chavkin, 1991).

One of the strongest objections to the use of pressure or coercion is the risk of driving women out of the health care system, particularly women who may have the greatest need for medical attention because of drug abuse or other risk factors.

Prosecution

No state has yet passed a law that provides for criminal prosecution on the basis of prenatal substance abuse. Although several states are considering such measures, it appears that the trend is away from consideration of punitive measures and toward the enactment of prevention and treatment measures and/or at least the development of task forces to further study the issue of what measures the legislature should pursue. A number of states are considering measures that would require the imposition of increased criminal penalties on an individual convicted of selling or distributing a controlled substance to a woman who is known to be pregnant (Marshall, 1991). So far, only one conviction has been upheld on appeal.

■□ SUMMARY

The best prevention is primary prevention, that is, to inform women of the dangers of alcohol and cocaine in pregnancy and for them to abstain during pregnancy. Teachers and service providers are most likely to be involved in primary prevention efforts, with new opportunities becoming available for early interventionists to do some secondary prevention. The concept of mothering from conception instead of from birth, rather than fear, should be emphasized. Providing information alone to women who are already involved with drugs and alcohol does little to change

behavior. Curricula based on social learning theory are more efficacious in changing behavior than fact-based curricula. The main barriers that keep women from seeking treatment are likely to be rooted
in the family and environment: stigma, opposition from family and
partner, and denial. Barriers that keep women out of treatment are lack
of child care, lack of transportation, lack of prenatal care in treatment
facilities, and lack of any available treatment. Mandatory treatment is
more likely to place disadvantaged women in incarceration rather than
treatment because good treatment facilities are unavailable. Mandatory treatment and prosecution are not viewed as good options. Ultimately, treatment capacity must be developed so that any drug-abusing woman who is pregnant or has young children and seeks treatment can receive treatment.

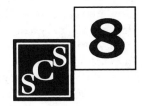

Children of Substance Abuse and P.L. 99-457: A Case for Program Evaluation

Part H (Public Law 99-457) was enacted in 1986 to deal with education of handicapped children under 3 years of age. Contrary to previous special education legislation, this law mandated the states to provide definitions of the children who will be served. At-risk children were designated as an optional category (VanBremen, 1991).

The states were given 5 years to develop plans to implement Part H and were given funding each year to further this process. Funding was contingent on approval of the states' plans. In the fourth year, states were required to submit their definitions of "developmentally delayed" and how it would be determined. Given the latitude in deciding which children would be included in coverage, definitions vary from state to state (VanBremen, 1991).

There is a consensus among those who work with children exposed prenatally to substances that P.L. 99-457 funds should be used to provide early intervention to children whose mothers used alcohol and/or illicit drugs while pregnant. The perspective of this book is clearly that many at-risk children exposed to substances respond well to early intervention, that is, parenting instruction for mothers and caregivers, regular evaluation of developmental needs, and enrollment in various kinds of therapy or early intervention programs. That perspective is supported by a small but growing body of research. It follows that these children should be included in the categories of children to be served under Part H. What we do not know is what kind of intervention works best: Should children exposed to drugs or alcohol be segregated into their own protected classrooms or mainstreamed? Are service providers most effective as collaborators or as therapists? Are home programs effective? How many visits should be planned to make a difference? What parenting skills translate to the best child outcome? What should we do to prepare FAS children to be productive adults? What educational programs are needed for personnel preparation? The list continues.

We are caught on the horns of a dilemma: We must show that early intervention is effective in order to obtain funding, but it is difficult to obtain funding for our programs until we show that they are effective. Unfortunately, many successful intervention programs do not provide enough program evaluation data for the stakeholders — administrators, policy makers, and funders — to be convinced of the seriousness of the problems exposed children face and of the efficacy of early intervention for them.

In this chapter, we will review the status of including children exposed to substances in the states' definitions for P.L. 99-457 and then review some methods for early intervention program evaluation that would be appropriate for programs serving children of substance abuse and their families. Cost analysis will be touched on briefly. Finally, a model program evaluation is described. The purpose of this discussion is to plant some ideas: Program evaluation is not scary; it is easier to do than we think; and it should be an integral part of every structured intervention program.

◾ P.L. 99-457: WHERE ARE WE?

VanBremen (1991) reviewed and analyzed, for the National Perinatal Addiction Research and Education (NAPARE), the states' definitions of categories of children to be served under Part H. To receive approval from the Office of Special Education (OSEP), states had to submit their definitions. States must serve children who are developmentally delay-ed or who have an established condition that leads to developmental delay. However, the states have the *option* of serving children who are at risk. There is great variation among states as to what is included in their definitions and in their decisions to include children at risk. "At-risk" is a particularly confusing term because some states have labeled establish-ed conditions as established risk, thus confusing this category with the optional at-risk category. It should also be noted that these definitions may be changed by the states as they begin to implement early interven-tion programs (VanBremen, 1991).

In addition to analyzing the definitions of states with OSEP ap-proval, VanBremen (1991) conducted a survey of all 50 states, asking for their current plans regarding the eligibility of children exposed to mater-nal substance abuse. Many states have not yet determined if maternal substance abuse will be included in the at-risk or established risk categories, if at all. Samples of these results with an example follow (VanBremen, 1991).

States with approved fourth-year funding definitions including maternal substance abuse as a criteria for eligibility. Hawaii includes infants born to mothers with a history of substance abuse in their fourth-year definition of biological risk. Eligibility in this category will be determined based on a statement signed by a physician, indicating the condition is likely to lead to developmental delay. Hawaii also elected to include in its eligible population children having two or more environmental risk factors. Ten risk factors are delineated, one of which is "abuse of any legal or illegal substance by a primary caregiver."

States with approved fourth-year definitions including maternal substance abuse with qualification. North Carolina lists parental substance ab-use as an indicator of high risk potential. Children with three such risk factors are eligible for services when accompanied by a pro-fessional determination of need for early intervention services.

States with fourth-year funding applications not including maternal sub-stance abuse. Colorado does not mention substance abuse as a con-dition associated with significant developmental delays in their fourth-year definition. The only criteria for determining eligibility of at-risk children are infants and toddlers who are children of parents with developmental disabilities. Although other children at risk for developmental delays are not included at this time, Colorado plans to study further other at-risk groups of children. Results of these studies may warrant expansion of the children eligible for services.

NAPARE's survey indicates that many states are responding to maternal substance abuse as an established risk factor that threatens normal infant and child development. However, even states that have decided to provide early intervention services to this group of children are under pressure to limit costs by restricting services. Service providers and other advocates for children prenatally exposed to drugs should express their views about the need to include this category in the eligibility definitions of their respective states (VanBremen, 1991).

■ PROGRAM EVALUATION

While the decision to include maternal substance abuse as a definition for early intervention is not made on the basis of empirical data alone, it is doubtful that maternal substance abuse will be included without some evidence of a causal link between substance abuse and risk for development. These linkages are now accepted. Our public values dictate that children who need service should receive it. The next question becomes, how can it be funded? It is at this point that another linkage must be shown: the efficacy of early intervention for such children and their families. Without good evidence of efficacy, "expensive, unevaluated programs that are continued year after year and that are based only on hunches and political winds can represent a waste of millions of dollars as well as lost opportunities to try what could well be more effective approaches" (Gomby & Larson, 1992, p. 68).

How, then, do we as service providers know which programs are effective with children exposed to maternal substances and which are no better, or perhaps worse, than regular education programs or no program at all? How do we approach the policy makers and funders with the conviction that we know what we are doing? For example, our programs for children exposed to drugs include a heavy component of family support, yet there are few studies on the best intensity level for family support programs, the types of caregivers that benefit from family support programs, or the amount of training that is appropriate for the home visitors who provide the family support (Roberts, Wasik, Casto, & Ramey, 1991). How disappointing it is to hear at professional meetings of programs or techniques about which the speaker is enthusiastic, but presents no evaluative data. How can I know if that program will be effective with the children and families that I work with?

Every school program or service effort should undergo some level of evaluation, whether for the purpose of honing an existing program or providing evidence of its effectiveness. Evaluation of our services is important for at least two reasons (Gomby & Larson, 1992).

1. Evaluation can provide information about whether the service approach is effective and/or worth the investment. Implementation of a new program for children exposed to drugs may require significant changes in funding and utilization of personnel and services. Such changes usually involve costs, and we should be able to demonstrate that the direct and indirect costs inherent in the program are warranted on the basis of demonstrated outcomes. Teachers and service providers want to know whether the changes they have made are improving the lives of children and families.

2. Evaluation can also provide information about how best to implement a program. An evaluation can be structured to help those implementing a program identify areas where they are meeting or exceeding goals or where the program should be modified to improve service to children and families.

Reluctance on the part of service providers and educators to build evaluation into their programs may stem from four reasons:

1. Evaluation is viewed as too hard to do. The only design seen as credible is the randomized experimental and control group which is expensive in both time and effort. The ideal of the true experimental design with standardized pre- and post-test measurements is difficult to achieve in program evaluation studies in general and may be impossible to achieve in Part H programs in particular. The ethics of using no-treatment control groups is increasingly being challenged, even though investigators argue that the effects of the treatment are only hypothesized and not known. As a consequence, some programs evaluate the comparative effectiveness of two different treatments. In the case of Part H programs, because services are made available to the entire population of those eligible, it may not be possible to identify an equivalent no-treatment group for comparison purposes (Murray, 1992).

2. Evaluation is viewed with suspicion. The arrival of outside evaluators to judge the worth of a program is threatening, the reports are often incomprehensible, and the results usually give

no indication to staff as to how the program could be improved (Murray, 1992). Providers worry that they will be held accountable for meeting unreasonable expectations regarding long-term, multifaceted problems. They fear that evaluators will focus on a narrow outcome (such as test scores) and overlook a less tangible but equally important change (such as improved cooperation among service providers). Service providers and planners fear that evaluators will get in the way by imposing, for the sake of the evaluation, such rigidity in a program that the main goal of serving children in a flexible and effective way will be thwarted (Gomby & Larson, 1992).

3. Unlike academicians, program staff are usually not interested in generalizations to other programs. Rather, they are interested in how their program works, what benefits their clients receive, and how their program can be improved. The majority of staff members at the local program level are trained as clinicians and have little personal experience, interest, or academic training in experimental design and statistical methods (Murray, 1992).

4. Monitoring efforts by Part H programs are presently hampered because a computer-based management information system designed specifically for early intervention programs is not available. Programming existing database or spreadsheet programs to do the job may require more time and expertise than most program staff have at their disposal (Murray, 1992).

■ TYPES OF EVALUATION

Evaluations are often divided into two general types, both of which can be useful in assessing Part H programs for at-risk children: process evaluations and outcome evaluations. In the following sections we will look at these two ways of evaluating programs for children exposed to substances. The first step in deciding which method to use is to determine the goals of the evaluation. Is the purpose of the evaluation to describe the services the program provided and who received them? Or is it to determine if and for whom the services made a difference?

Process Evaluation

Process evaluations, or formative evaluations, focus on what services were provided to whom and how. Their purpose is to describe how the program was implemented — who was involved and what problems were experienced. A process evaluation is useful for monitoring program implementation; for identifying changes to make the program operate as planned; and, generally, for program improvement (Gomby & Larson, 1992). It is essential to know whether the project could be carried out as originally planned. Often programs previously established as successful in demonstration projects are found to be ineffective because they were diluted when implemented on a wide scale. For example, instead of two home visits per month, staff may be able to manage only one home visit every 6 weeks because of limited budgets. A diluted program would not be expected to have the same impact as the fully implemented program (Murray, 1992). That problem would become evident in a process evaluation.

Outcome Evaluation

Outcome evaluations, or summative evaluations, are studies to determine the effectiveness or outcomes of a program. They must be designed to measure whether the anticipated changes occurred and to prove that the changes were caused by the program and not something else, that is, that the program caused the change. For example, test scores may increase after a program is introduced, but this information alone cannot prove that the program caused the change. Unlike process evaluation results, outcome evaluation results may generalize beyond the particular program evaluated and suggest what models may be effective in other sites. Outcome evaluations are usually related to child-centered goals, such as academic performance or reduction in challenging behaviors. An outcome evaluation can be undertaken if there are clear goals about what changes are expected and appropriate measures are selected for tracking the changes. As a general rule, to help establish a causal link between the provided services and observed changes and to eliminate alternative explanations of outcomes, evaluators must compare students or families who did not receive the services with similar students who did. Researchers often use one of two techniques to construct a comparison group (Gomby & Larson, 1992):

1. Match the group (such as students, classrooms, or schools) receiving services with a similar group that does not receive services.
2. Use random assignment to decide which members of a target group receive services and which do not.

Qualitative and Quantitative Methods

In the traditional quantitative approach, variables and outcomes are specified in advance, measured in operational quantities, and subjected to experimental manipulations that are measured in some way. An hypothesis is formed and statistical significance is evaluated. Important variables are identified before data collections begin. Output measures may be posttest measures after an intervention, new skills, or costs. The quantitative approach depends on breaking the program system into several parts. The qualitative approach is more holistic. Important variables emerge as the program goes on. The investigator studies what occurs in the program without trying to control, manipulate, or artificially interrelate what happens.

Murray (1992) argues that Part H early intervention programs would be better served by qualitative, rather than quantitative, evaluation methods. Qualitative approaches seek not to predict and generalize, but rather to understand. The approach seeks to understand the subjective reality of program participants, their perceptions and judgments, rather than to obtain objective numeric scores. The user of qualitative methods carries out naturalistic observations and open-ended interview procedures. This contrasts with quantitative analysis, which requires segmentation for the purpose of measuring component parts or isolating single causal variables. An example of qualitative evaluation was provided in Chapter 3 when a group of mothers and a group of professionals were asked to describe the behavior of infants and toddlers.

Qualitative data are basically detailed descriptions that can consist of notes of observations made during visits to a program, verbatim transcripts of what was said during interviews with staff or participants, or copies of documents or reports kept in participants' files. Rather than statistical analysis, a content analysis is used to analyze the data. In a purely qualitative study, there are no preconceived hypotheses, no large random samples, no manipulation of treatment conditions, no standardized measures, and no inferential statistical analysis.

Despite the heavy family focus of programs for children exposed to maternal substances, there are few accepted, that is, standardized, measures of family support and family functioning (Black, 1991; Roberts et al., 1991). The research-based instruments that are available typically were not developed for clinical use and are often found offensive and intrusive by parents (Murray, 1992). As pointed out in Chapter 9, many clinical instruments likewise are inappropriate for use in research; and as was pointed out in Chapter 3, using standardized developmental assessments with children exposed to maternal substances does not give a true picture of their performance or behavior. Thus, quantitative measures for developmental outcome assessments are not available for Part H programs that serve infants and toddlers exposed to maternal substances. According to Murray (1992), "Indeed the heterogeneity of the population targeted, the individualized nature of the services provided, and the variability of the expected outcomes for each case preclude the use of standardized measures for impact assessment" (p. 81).

An alternative to quantification of child outcomes based on standardized measures includes goal attainment scaling, a method of tracking progress toward individualized goals (Murray, 1992).

Qualitative methods appear to be particularly suited to the individualized family-centered approach that is the basis of the Part H legislation. Because the population of children served is extremely heterogeneous with respect to developmental disorders, and because service plans are individualized and developed with the active participation of families, uniform outcomes are not expected. Therefore, standardized assessments are not appropriate for documenting program effects. The lack of uniformity across children and treatments will make these programs a nightmare for those who wish to conduct quantitative outcome studies. Thus a case study approach is more suited to the philosophy and delivery of Part H infant and toddler services (Murray, 1992).

A feature of the Part H programs that meshes well with qualitative evaluation methods is that assessments and service plans are intended to be holistic rather than segmenting the child into component parts. The emergence of techniques for transdisciplinary play assessments is evidence of this holistic approach. In this approach, a single professional on a team facilitates play so that the team can observe the behaviors required to judge the child's skill level in many areas. In recognition of the inadequacy of traditional norm-referenced tests, many early interventionists are turning to judgment-based assessments, which can be used to tap the clinical judgment of professionals as well as to integrate the family into the assessment process (Bagnato & Neisworth, 1991).

Another reason for using qualitative methods of evaluation is that the methods used by staff and evaluators are similar. For example, many Part H programs include home visits, which put the early interventionist in the role of participant observer. With little training, staff can keep notes that can be used later to write case studies for an implementation evaluation. An evaluator can assist in developing an interview guide to obtain the needed information in a relaxed, in-depth interview. Transcripts or notes based on these interviews can provide the information needed for writing the Individualized Family Service Plan (IFSP) as well as the raw data for a qualitative analysis of family needs, so that gaps in services can be identified and filled (Murray, 1992).

Qualitative Evaluation Methods

Methods include participant observation, in-depth interviewing, group interviews, and case studies.

Participant Observation

When used for program evaluation, participant observation involves a combination of observation and interview of key informants during the normal operation of the program. Informants might include parents, teachers, caregivers, or service providers. What transpired while visiting a program is immediately documented in field notes. The notes are rich in descriptive detail and include as much of the informants' own words as possible. Interpretations made by the evaluator are clearly marked as separate from the descriptive material. At the outset, the qualitative evaluator has no preconceived ideas or categories defined *a priori* for observation. Rather, the categories are developed *a posteriori* from the data during the course of the study and are finalized during the final analysis phase of the project (Murray, 1992).

In-Depth Interviewing

In-depth interviews are conducted in addition to the casual interviews conducted during participant observation. The interviewer may have a list of general topic areas to cover or even specific questions to ask, but the answers to the questions are open-ended. This contrasts to the more structured questionnaires or interviews that provide multiple-choice or closed-response categories for ease of quantification. Transcripts of the interviews are analyzed for content by means of a general procedure of sorting through the comments to classify them according to higher order concepts and to establish linkages between concepts (Mirriam, 1988).

Group Interviews (Focus Groups)

Focus groups are being used increasingly in evaluation research. The typical focus group brings together a homogeneous group of 6 to 10 participants for about a 2-hour discussion. The group leader guides the discussion with a carefully prepared set of approximately six to eight questions called the questioning route. The session is audiotaped so that verbatim transcripts of the discussion can be prepared and the comments are analyzed for content.

Murray (1992) cites an example of the use of focus groups for Part H planning. Summers, Dell'Oliver, and Turnbull (1990) conducted eight focus groups of parents and professionals to obtain opinions about the IFSP process and outcomes. A major outcome of the study was the finding that participants strongly objected to the use of standardized family assessment measures and preferred informal and unintrusive (i.e., qualitative) methods such as open-ended conversations likened to the telling of stories. Another major finding was that families viewed the early intervention practitioner's role more as provider of emotional support and friendship rather than a knowledgeable expert. Thus the families valued interdependence over the concept of independence and empowerment. The IFSP approach has been recommended in this book both for families affected by alcohol and by cocaine for various reasons, the most obvious being Part H guidelines. It would be interesting to see if the same result would be obtained if the focus group consisted of women in a comprehensive treatment program with their children or women in the later stages of recovery who are learning parenting skills.

Case Studies

Case studies are in-depth descriptions of individual cases designed to highlight their unique features. These cases may represent individual program participants or entire programs. For example, a process evaluation may consist of a detailed study of a few participants to document and understand how the program is experienced personally by participants. It could also compare cases of participants who clearly benefitted with those who did not benefit from the program (Murray, 1992). It should be noted that the case studies in this book are not useful for program evaluation, because the children did not receive the same program. Rather they are stories of real children used as illustrations of children exposed to maternal alcohol and cocaine.

Cost Analysis

As we approach funders with our data on program evaluation, we should also have an idea of the costs of the program. There are several different types of cost analyses, and their methods of computation will not be discussed here. However, it is beneficial to know what values are in the numerator and denominator of the most common types of cost analyses.

1. *Cost effectiveness or cost efficiency* (C/E = > 1). This analysis is done after a program is completed. The program objectives are divided by the actual resources that were spent. For example, 10 families were served at a cost of $5,000. The cost effectiveness was $500 per family.
2. *Cost feasibility* (C/budget = < 1). How much budget is available for the cost of the program? The projected cost of the program is $3,000 and the budget is $5,000. The cost is feasible because $3,000/$5,000 = less than 1.
3. *Cost benefit* (B/C = > 1). What is the benefit to a person in the program, perhaps for his or her lifetime? This is the type of analysis that is done to show the benefit of saving a life or graduating from school. The benefit may include the total lifetime earnings of that person divided by the cost of the program. Total benefit can never be accurately calculated. (How can quality of life be reduced to monetary terms?) As an example, the projected cost of a special vocational counselor for 10 FAS high school students is $35,000 per year. The FAS students would then be expected to earn $10,000 per year more than they would have earned without the counselor. $100,000/$35,000 = more than 1 for the first year, considerably more if an average lifespan is considered.

A Program Evaluation Model: The Schools in Communities Program, New York State

The following is a comprehensive community- and school-based program that required considerable planning and commitment of resources. It is included here to illustrate the evaluation methods that were used. Some of the methods could be used with considerably fewer resources.

This state initiative began in January 1987, with community schools programs in four school districts participating. In fiscal year 1991-1992 there will be 33 community schools programs statewide. The program is based on the conviction that all children can learn and that a strong school-community partnership is essential to achieve this goal. The primary goal of the program is to improve student outcomes by providing comprehensive education, health, nutrition, and other support services required by students and families.

Program Description

To provide a framework of expectations for each school, the New York State Board of Regents identified 15 characteristics desired for the Schools in Communities Program. To implement the characteristics and to achieve the program's major objectives, the New York State Education Department determined that a number of program and budgetary requirements must be met. Within these requirements, each district has flexibility in how it addresses the unique needs of its own community.

The program requirements include availability of services on an extended day, week, and year basis; a full-day prekindergarten program; a full-time community schools program coordinator; a management planning team that includes the coordinator; an advisory committee that includes parents and community members; effective involvement of parents; and the establishment of service linkages (on-site, if possible) with public and private agencies, community-based organizations, colleges, businesses, and cultural and religious institutions.

The budgetary requirements include submission of annual budgets and final fiscal reports; a dollar-for-dollar match of state funds by the local school district; and a commitment by the district to seek third-party funding sources to support and expand services.

Evaluation Methods

The nature of the evaluation has changed over the 4 years since the program began. From the beginning, each school was required to submit a yearly report about the progress it had made in meeting goals and about the problems encountered. Each school's report is now a comprehensive, annual evaluation composed of:

- ◼ *A baseline report* submitted by each grantee at the beginning of funding. This report identifies services and achievements in the year prior to Schools in Communities funding. This determines a base against which future data can be evaluated.
- ◼ *An annual evaluation report.* This report details the services offered; the number of students and families served; and the progress of the program during the year, as measured against program objectives.
- ◼ *A monitoring report* completed on-site by teams from the state Education Department. This report is submitted to the district superintendent, who is given an opportunity to respond.

In addition, assigned staff from the state Education Department visit each site regularly to provide technical assistance and to monitor progress.

Annually, the state Education Department submits a comprehensive program report to the Board of Regents. The report presents the data gathered during the year and is intended to show progress in making schools the nucleus of service for their communities. It also indicates the uniqueness of approaches determined by each school and district to meet its identified needs. This report is available to the public.

Achieving improvement in measures of outcomes, such as achievement test scores, dropout rates, and attendance rates is a primary long-range goal of the New York State Education Department (*The Future of Children*, 1992).[1]

The parts of this evaluation divided into outcome and process evaluation are shown in Table 8–1. Two important messages for school personnel are:

TABLE 8-1

Differences between outcome evaluations and process evaluations

Description	Outcome Evaluation	Process Evaluation
Purpose	Meeting goals	Documenting problems encountered
Data and reports	Comparison groups	Annual reports include
	Baseline—data from prior year	Services offered
	Compare annual report data to baseline	Number of students and families participating
	Report to State Board shows goals	Monitoring reports— ongoing
	Achievement test scores	
	Drop-out rates	
	Attendance	

[1] For further information on this program, the contact person is Lester W. Young, Jr., Associate Commissioner, Office of School and Community Services, New York State Education Department, 55 Hanson Place, Room 400, Brooklyn, NY 11217, (718) 260-2796.

1. Keep process evaluation data from the inception of your program: numbers of students and families served; nature of the services; how progress was made; how the program was perceived by those doing it and those receiving it, such as staff and parents (drug using, recovering, and non-drug using); problems encountered and changes made.
2. If possible, do an outcome evaluation by comparing predetermined outcome measures in a treated and an untreated group. Those measures could include: attendance, transition to preschool or school, parenting skills, parent satisfaction, or child achievement.

■ SUMMARY

Every program for children exposed to prenatal substance abuse should have an evaluation component from its inception. Evaluations need not require an onerous commitment of resources. With little additional effort and with the assistance of either an in-house evaluator or a consultant, qualitative data can be systematically collected by staff of Part H programs. This information can be used for both decision-making regarding individual clients and as raw data for a content analysis in process evaluation. Although outcome evaluations usually are quantitative, qualitative data can also be used in evaluations of program impact when it is possible to identify distinct comparison groups (i.e., participants exposed to different program models). On the basis of program evaluation, we can look at intervention programs objectively and convince policy makers and funders that these at-risk children should be included in Part H funding.

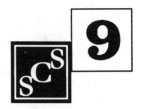

Research in Substance Abuse

he focus of this book has been on providing services for children, who have been prenatally exposed to substances, in early intervention and school programs. It would seem that a chapter on research, then, would be misplaced. However, service providers and educators faced with the problem of designing interventions for children who have been exposed to drugs prenatally are understandably calling for good research on which to base their interventions. Much of the current literature presents conflicting results regarding the type and magnitude of the impact of prenatal substance abuse. An understanding of the problems involved in investigations of prenatal substance exposure helps explain these inconsistent findings and the limitations of our knowledge (Zuckerman, 1991). Furthermore, service providers and researchers are not mutually exclusive. There is a need for clinical research with solid research methodology.

In this chapter, the research process and attendant methodologic issues in conducting infant behavioral research when maternal substance use is a variable of interest will be discussed. The purpose of the discussion is not to direct the reader in how to do research; rather it is to point out, based on my own experience, cautions about methodology when substance use is involved. The research project described here was hospital-based, but school-based researchers may find that they face some of the same problems. (Readers interested in methodology are referred to Chasnoff, 1991a.)

The bare essentials of my research question will help to understand that process. The project, conducted in a teaching hospital in a medium-sized city, used a quasi-experimental research design; that is, an experiment that has treatments, outcome measures, and experimental units, but does not use random assignment (Cook & Campbell, 1979). The experimental group consisted of all infants born during a 1-year period whose mothers had used cocaine during pregnancy and who would consent to have their infants in the study. The control group included infants matched for birth weight, race, and other maternal drug history, but without prenatal cocaine exposure. The specific aim of the study was to measure differences in interactions between experimental and control group infants. The measurements were taken during the first week of life and again at 2 months of age. Our research team consisted of the author as principal investigator from the university (outside investigator) and a pediatrician and a nurse on staff at the hospital (inside investigators).

◼◻ RESEARCH PROCESS

Certain steps are common to all research: (1) choosing the problem and stating the hypothesis, (2) formulating the research design, (3) data collection, (4) coding and analyzing data, and (5) interpreting results. Since interpretations of results stimulate new research problems, the process forms a continuous loop (Bailey, 1978). Although all good research is difficult and demands a serious commitment in time and talent, research in the area of substance abuse poses distinct challenges that will be discussed at each step of the research process.

◼◻ THE PROBLEM AND HYPOTHESIS

Benefits vs. Exploitation

Testing the hypothesis is, of course, the essence of quantative research. In research related to substance abuse, it is especially important for study results to have clear benefits for the study population. The least one should do as an investigator is to guard against actual harm; the best is to benefit others in the target population as an outcome of the research. Those who choose to conduct research in the emotionally charged milieu of drug use must be prepared not only to fulfill the letter and spirit of human subjects' protections, but also to guard against any exploitation, or appearance of exploitation, of subjects. In other words, the reasons for asking women to disclose what substances they used while they were pregnant should be clear to them and to others.

The project team must be prepared to counter any perception of exploitation before it surfaces from others whose cooperation is essential to the success of the project: attending physicians, staff nurses, social workers, and one's colleagues (or analagous school personnel, if the research is conducted there). In this study, the project nurse found it helpful periodically to discuss the research in nursing staff meetings and answer questions, as did the pediatrician in her unit meetings. I also was careful to focus on the positive outcome when discussing the project with colleagues and friends; for example, "We are looking at the interactions of babies when their mothers have taken cocaine so that we can help the babies to develop."

■ RESEARCH DESIGN

Three issues warrant particular attention in designing a substance use study: control for polydrug exposure, selection of a representative sample, and inclusion of sufficient numbers to be confident of a main effect. The latter two problems are faced in every research design but have some twists in a substance abuse design that need consideration. The former, however, is unique to research in this population.

Control for Polydrug Use

Research on a drug's subsequent effects on children is challenging because drug-dependent women rarely use just one drug. It is especially difficult to design research to control for polydrug use. Illegal drugs, such as cocaine, methamphetamines, PCP, and marijuana, are commonly combined with alcohol and cigarettes. This pattern of polydrug use, coupled with the fact that the illegal substances ingested are seldom pure, makes it difficult to determine which drugs a pregnant woman has used, when they were used during pregnancy, and how much of a drug (or drugs) she has taken. In addition, drug-dependent, pregnant women often have poor nutrition, are subject to increased infections and other medical complications, and receive little or no prenatal care. All of these factors can cause problems for infants, making it difficult to separate the effects of drugs from the effects of a generally unhealthy prenatal environment or maternal lifestyle (Kronstadt, 1992).

One design that can be used to control for this problem is a matched cohort study. Infants or children are matched to be alike in all variables except the variable under investigation, such as the main effect of cocaine or alcohol. In our study, subjects were matched for race, sex, birth weight (within 8 oz), and socioeconomic status. However, the more variables matched, the more limited is the pool of control subjects. Our variable of interest was cocaine exposure or no cocaine exposure. That meant we wanted control mothers to have used other drugs, such as marijuana and alcohol, because the cocaine-using mothers also used those drugs.

When the purpose of a study is to determine the main effect of a particular drug, it is crucial to have a control group in which that drug was not used at any time during the pregnancy. How would we determine that our control group mothers had not used cocaine? We used three controls for polydrug use: urine screens on mother and infant, meconium testing of infants, and drug histories on the mothers. None of these is a completely objective and reliable measure.

Urine Toxicology Screens

Urine screens measure a concentration of the cocaine metabolite in the urine that remains in the mother's body for approximately 48 hours after use. However, if the mother drinks enough water to dilute her urine, the concentration of the metabolite in her urine will fall below the laboratory threshold for a positive report. Newborn urine is relatively diluted in the first 24 hours, hence the concentration of the metabolite may fall below the standard threshold for the baby as well. Moreover, urine screens were not done on every mother and infant, only on suspicion of drug use. Suspicion consisted of (a) no prenatal care and (b) a prior history of drug use. When a positive urine toxicology screen for cocaine was found on either the mother or the infant, the mother was considered a possible experimental group subject who could be approached to grant her informed consent to participate in the study. The control group mothers were more of a challenge. We recruited our matched control subjects from mothers who had not had a drug screen or who had had a screen that was positive for marijuana but not cocaine. We assumed that at least some of the mothers in the latter group had, in fact, used cocaine in pregnancy and had remained undetected because they were either not screened or the screen did not detect the metabolite. If we included these subjects in our control group and they had indeed used cocaine, our results would be in error. We needed to have a test other than the mother's self-report of her drug use and decided to analyze meconium on both experimental and control infants.

Meconium Testing

As discussed in Chapter 3, a more sensitive test to determine if a neonate has been exposed to any of four drugs (cocaine, heroin, marijuana, and amphetamines) during gestation is available in which a first stool specimen (meconium) is analyzed. This method is not error-free, however, as we discovered when a report for one of the infants whose mother reported high dosages of cocaine throughout her pregnancy came back negative. We blamed human error in collecting the sample. The meconium test served as a first test of drug use for the control group and as corroboration for the experimental group.

Mothers' Drug Histories

Neither urine nor meconium tests report the amount of the drug used, only if the concentration of the metabolite is sufficient to cross the test threshold. This limitation has impeded the establishment of dose-effect relationships for outcomes associated with cocaine use. A difficult problem of research in prenatal exposure to various chemical substances is the need to rely on subjects' reports of their own behavior in this emotionally charged area. Naturally women may under-report their use of illegal or socially stigmatized substances (Zuckerman, 1991). We took careful histories of drug use, including amount used, method of administration, and timing of use, all of which have room for error (Chasnoff, 1991a).

- ◼ *Amount.* The concentration of cocaine may vary from one community to another and may vary within a community.
- ◼ *Administration.* The drug under study, although labeled "cocaine," may take many forms and may be used in different ways: inhaled, smoked, free-based, or injected.
- ◼ *Timing.* The dose of cocaine used can vary for the individual user or over a particular time frame, as in the 40 weeks of pregnancy.

Researchers naive to the use of street drugs are well advised to rely on questionnaires devised for drug histories found in drug-abuse treatment facilities, and then modify them for their own use and coding system. My first few drug histories were revelations in terminology. The experimental group mothers seemed to be forthcoming about their drug use; it was, after all, now a known fact. Two mothers told me (and it was verified by a drug counselor) that a *primo* is a rock of crack (cocaine) smoked with marijuana, and primos were by far the preferred method of administration by the cocaine-using mothers in my study. This posed a methodological problem: How to control for marijuana use when finding the main effect of cocaine? It became even more important for the control group to include matched cohorts for marijuana use. One mother said she used primos but *not* marijuana. Could she be unaware that primos contain marijuana? She also denied crack use, although her hospital chart documented that she admitted using crack and four previous children had been removed from her care because of her crack use. She said she smoked cocaine powder in a pipe in the first two trimesters and switched to primos, which she called cocaine powder and tobacco, in the last trimester. Obviously, there is considerable room for measurement error in the histories, and we had to make every effort to verify the substance used, dosage, and timing by going over the history at both the birth and the infant's 2-month testing.

Selecting the Sample

The target population is children exposed prenatally to a substance. The sample, then, should be representative of that population. If the sample is drawn too narrowly, results from that sample will not generalize (or be externally valid) to other children exposed to the same drug. Generalization is threatened by the way the samples of children are chosen in most studies of children exposed to substances. The setting of the project also can affect the recruitment of study subjects and, thus, the definition of the population under study. In this study, where children were primarily black and of low socioeconomic status, results can be generalized only to other exposed children who are black and of the same status. In fact, according to Chasnoff, Landress, and Barrett (1990), our present knowledge of prenatal drug exposure is based mainly on information gathered from indigent, nonwhite women and their children. Although substance abuse during pregnancy cuts across all socioeconomic classes and ethnic groups, it is usually the poor and women who are identified as substance abusers and, therefore, come to the attention of service providers and researchers. We do not know if the effects attributed to drug use would be observed among more well-to-do families who, with additional resources, might be able to cushion the effects of drug exposure on their children (Kronstadt, 1991). Chasnoff et al. (1992), caution against generalizing their results to all drug-exposed children when their study population comprises mothers who had good prenatal care and were motivated to stop their drug use during pregnancy.

It is vitally important that the control group be demographically comparable to the experimental group. Some studies use an experimental group of drug-exposed children and a comparison group of nonexposed children without reporting sufficient information concerning the characteristics of the control group to know if the groups are comparable; all we know is that the control group mothers did not use drugs. The investigators could have compared mothers who received prenatal care with those who did not, white mothers with black mothers, or inner city children with suburban children — all of which would introduce error into the study. Although a control group may be demographically similar to the group under study, there is little one can do to control for the drug-seeking environment in which most of the women and their children under study live (Chasnoff, 1991b). The effects of the environment will be more compelling as a child gets older, thus making the comparability of groups even more doubtful.

Particularly disturbing are studies, seen all too often in the literature, in which drug-exposed children who are in intervention programs are compared to some standardized test norm, or even to a group of children who are not in intervention, and the study results are interpreted to mean that the drug-exposed children have deficits of certain kinds. If the experimental group is chosen from children receiving intervention, it cannot be a surprise that they have deficits. Children who are not in intervention programs are not included in the study experimental groups. The point cannot be overemphasized: Not all children exposed prenatally to drugs or alcohol will have deficits. Results based on such biased sampling can only be considered spurious.

Sufficient Numbers of Subjects

To ensure that our sample is representative, we must have sufficient numbers of subjects in each group. We must ask the question: Are there enough cases in the study to ensure that the results have a reasonable chance of being true or have we sampled only extreme cases? Unfortunately, we usually are confined to the population that walks in a particular door, whether it is a school, a clinic, or a drug rehabilitation facility, and have access not to a random sample but a convenience sample. The numbers must be sufficiently large in a convenience sample to lessen the threat to generalizability. However, in the real world, our sample generally is determined by how much money we have to spend on sampling, particularly if the subjects are paid. For more about sufficient numbers, see Cohen (1977).

◼ DATA COLLECTION

Data collection from drug users and former users poses a number of problems: gaining access to the population, gaining cooperation of the mothers, and using valid and reliable instruments to measure outcome variables.

Kelly (1979) describes research settings as being *responsive* or *resistant* to the researcher. He suggests researcher skills that are important to facilitate a responsive environment: (a) developing an active working relationship with influential persons, which involves expressing appropriate etiquettes and courtesies, and (b) creating alliances. Influential persons who have direct access to the site and target population are termed "gatekeepers" (Bloom, 1981). Gatekeepers in a large hospital can be divided into three groups: (a) those giving access to the site, such as the institutional review board; (b) those with access to the population, such as physicians; and (c) those within the institution who have day-to-day contact with the population, such as nurses.

Gaining Access to the Population

The Institutional Review Board (IRB)

Research concerning maternal substance abuse involves not only human subjects, but very sensitive ethical, psychological, and political issues. For example, uncovering drug use may result in severe repercussions for the mother, such as removal of the child from the home and/or criminal prosecution in the case of cocaine. When the substance is alcohol, guilt feelings and stigmatization may ensue. Consideration of their duty to protect human subjects must be weighed against the merits of a researcher's proposal by the IRB. With two institutions involved, I needed to have the approval of the IRB of my own university, as well as approval of the IRB of the hospital, before any funding source could be approached or any pilot testing could be done to test the protocol. I was caught in a dilemma: to decide if access should be given, the IRBs wanted a full and detailed proposal. However, I did not know if a newborn could respond to the protocol as I had designed it, and I could not try it on any newborns in the hospital until a full proposal, including the protocol, was approved.

Furthermore, the university IRB and the hospital IRB quite appropriately had different approaches to the proposal reflecting the constituencies of the two institutions. The university IRB was primarily interested in preserving the anonymity of the mothers, which meant strict confidentiality of data. The hospital IRB was concerned that individual infants would not receive appropriate treatment if the researcher had information about an infant's drug status and did not inform the infant's physician. The process of approval from both boards took 9 months of negotiating and required compromises on both sides. Points of negotiation were: Where are data to be stored, and how long should it be retained? Who has access to the data? How would confidentiality be maintained? How would the study be reported? What should be included in the informed consent? Would either institution be liable in any way?

Physicians

Collaboration between institutions on a research proposal may be instigated by investigators from each of the institutions who are acquainted, find an idea of interest, and decide to pursue it together; or the idea might originate with an investigator in one institution who must find a collaborator within the other institution. My project required that I find a collaborator within the hospital who would also be co-investigator, who could track the birth of infants exposed to cocaine, and had access to control group infants in the newborn nursery. Such a collaborator would also bring knowledge and experience that would be important to the project.

For the researcher who is an outsider, some history with the institution can help to aid alliances that lead to collaboration: past work on community enterprises in cooperation with physicians or attendance at educational programs at the hospital whereby the physicians have become acquainted with the investigators. Sometimes personal contacts have not been made previously, and the investigator must stand on his or her credibility as a researcher. I began by asking the advice of a physician on the staff with whom I was acquainted. He suggested the pediatrician who became the co-investigator of the project. I simply called her and explained my proposal. She was interested and, in turn, obtained permission from her supervisor. This hospital encourages research by staff physicians, especially those physicians who are involved with resident training.

The internal co-investigator became a partner in every sense of the word. Although the original design, including outcome measures and data analysis, was my responsibility, the project was shaped considerably from the beginning by her input. She had complete understanding of the goals of the project and was willing to devote time and energy to the project although she received no compensation for her time. Her involvement was also crucial to the institutional review board process; no longer did the project come from outside, but a staff physician was also involved who appeared with me at the hospital's IRB meetings.

Nurses

A metropolitan hospital, where my research was conducted, is a busy place where the primary focus is not to provide a milieu for the conduct of social research from a university. The appropriate etiquettes and courtesies assume particular importance. It goes without saying that scrupulous adherence to hospital rules and sanitary protocols is necessary. The nursing staff became accustomed to my presence in the nursery. Whenever I planned to have contact with a baby, I scrubbed and wore a gown. Although I often had to ask questions of the nurses, I was careful not to interfere with their routines.

Central to our project was the knowledge that a baby had been born who had a positive urine test for cocaine, or whose mother had a positive urine test. The nursery nurses had the first knowledge of those tests. The physician co-investigator was successful in recruiting a unit nurse to work on the project. Her involvement was absolutely crucial to the data-gathering process. She was responsible for reminding the other nurses to inform her if a baby positive for cocaine was born. She most often made the first contact with the mother to explain the project and gain informed consent, and she scheduled the measurement sessions. She received hospital scale payment per hour for her participation.

Gaining Cooperation of the Mothers

Considerable responsibility for the project's success rests with the mothers. They must sign an informed consent which states that they understand the purpose of the research and agree to a number of conditions: They must give an accounting of their drug use during pregnancy; they must allow the baby to be a subject for the protocol; and they must bring the baby back to the hospital at age 2 months to complete the protocol.

The first few minutes with a mother were crucial. We had to introduce ourselves and explain in a sentence or two what the study was about in a nonthreatening way and interject that mothers were paid for their time when they brought the baby back for the second visit. In the negotiations concerning informed consent, both the hospital and the university added or changed language in the informed consent form, spelling out confidentiality and liability. The result was a two-page document, much of which was written in convoluted and legalistic style, that one of us painstakingly reviewed with each mother.

The surprise in this process was the relative ease of obtaining consent from the cocaine-positive mothers, compared to the extreme difficulty in obtaining consent from potential control group subjects. As stated previously, we approached cocaine-positive mothers after the hospital's urine toxicology test came back positive and the mother had been so informed; at that point her drug use was known. The fact that we would then take a stool specimen from the baby for drug analysis was only confirmatory. However, the control infants were chosen from newborns in the nursery who matched the experimental group newborns, who had not had a urine screen, or who had a negative screen. Therefore, there was some doubt about the drug status of the mother; she could have used cocaine but not been screened; she could have used cocaine at some time during the pregnancy and the screen did not detect it; or she could be drug free. When these mothers were approached, they were told the purpose of the study and that if they chose to participate, a stool specimen would be taken for laboratory analysis. The specimen would report if the mother had used cocaine anytime after the first trimester of pregnancy. It was at this juncture that many of our possible control group mothers backed out. Time after time, mothers of potential control group subjects seemed interested until we asked for a drug screen and drug history. Some of these mothers said no immediately. Others made an appointment for a time after they left the hospital and then did not appear.

Incentives and Disincentives for Cooperation

Based on conversations with these mothers, their reasons for nonparticipation seemed to be (a) they had used cocaine during the pregnancy and they feared detection and (b) they feared reprisal for use of other drugs. Although we offered monetary incentives, the disincentives were too high.

Detection could mean removal of the baby by Social Services. In the first months of the study, our experimental group babies went home with their mothers and the mothers brought them back for the follow-up. However, during the study, the hospital procedure changed so that cocaine-exposed infants were removed by Protective Services and placed in foster care. In a few cases an infant was removed before we were aware of the positive cocaine screen and a potential experimental baby was lost to us. The political climate in the state as it pertained to punitive measures for prenatal substance use had changed also; two mothers in other cities were charged with the criminal offense of delivery of a controlled substance (cocaine) to the fetus and the charges received considerable publicity. The charges were dismissed by the judges as being outside the spirit of the law on delivery of cocaine. However, in such a climate, our assurance of confidentiality and the promise of financial reimbursement seemed to make little difference.

The positive effect of remuneration on response rate (Bryant, Kovar, & Miller, 1975) appears to be substantiated in this project. All of the mothers in the experimental group returned for follow-up, some even in the face of adverse circumstances, such as bringing several other children along and having to ask others for transportation. The response rate of the control mothers, given the same incentive, was not as high. Whatever reprisals experimental group mothers experienced were not dependent on their participation in our study, and the financial incentive would seem to be operative without a counter-incentive. Conversely, the experimental group would seem to have little reason, other than financial reward, for participation.

■□ VALID AND RELIABLE INSTRUMENTS FOR OUTCOME MEASURES

According to Kronstadt (1991), the tools we have to assess child development are problematical. Standardized developmental assessment tests may not be sensitive enough to pick up subtle variations in learning and behavior of children prenatally exposed to drugs. The tests may not be able to capture the elusive indicators that can predict later learning problems for substance-exposed children. Even if differences are observed, we do not always know the functional significance of the differences. For many tests, the extent to which the test results are useful predictors for subsequent performance in the real world (e.g., in school, in jobs) is unknown.

■□ CODING AND ANALYZING DATA

It is beyond the scope of this book to discuss methods for analyzing data. However, a word of caution is warranted under this topic: Those who do the data collection, whether it is from a checklist or from a standardized instrument, *must* be unaware of the drug-exposed status of the child being scored. Examiner bias is a major source of error. Many of the studies discussed in Chapter 3 did not use so called "blind" observers. In this study, it proved to be impossible to have the examiner blind to the infant's group designation; however, the interactions were recorded on videotape, and those who did the actual coding for analysis did not know if the infant they saw on the tape was drug-exposed or not.

■□ INTERPRETATION OF RESULTS

Because of the difficulties discussed briefly here, we should almost expect to see differing results from studies purporting to address the same question. Reconciling conflicting results requires that we be able to identify who was studied, the methods that the researchers used to ascertain what drugs were taken, and the tests used to find the reported developmental problems in the children. Variation between studies in any one of these factors could lead to differing results. When differences are found, we should consider their magnitude and their functional meaning in determining their importance (Kronstadt, 1991).

■□ OTHER CONSIDERATIONS

Any researcher will recognize that certain nonscientific practices are also involved in conducting research. One must identify sources of funding, arrange for adequate research space, and attend to many other logistical concerns. Although these activities merely support the basic scientific endeavor, they are essential to its success (Snowden, Munoz, & Kelly, 1979). Although not specific to substance use research, of particular importance is the commitment of time and energy of the research team to the project.

As our project progressed, each of the three project staff members had to renew her commitment to the project. The time commitment was the most daunting, especially for the nurse who scheduled appointments. Most of the mothers did not have telephones, so reminder letters for appointments had to be sent out. If a mother had a telephone, the nurse called the mother the night before and the morning of the appointment. Even so, missed appointments and consequent rescheduling were onerous. Our project was funded for only 1 year, and we had the expected interferences: other commitments by all three project staff, including family crises, illnesses, and vacations. To renew our commitment, the three of us needed to keep in touch with the aspects of the project and with each other. We had periodic meetings every 2 months to reestablish goals for each of us and review our database, including numbers of subjects and missing data.

■□ SUMMARY

Methodologic issues involved in the study of the impact of substances on developmental outcomes of children prenatally exposed to drugs have hampered study interpretations and development of appropriate interventions. Polydrug exposure and risks attendant to the lifestyle of the drug user make attributing developmental effects to one particular drug very suspicious. Other issues of concern in interpreting studies in this population are small sample sizes and lack of comparable control groups. Future research should examine development of substance-exposed children in larger and more varied groups and in a variety of environments, including stable, nurturant home conditions.

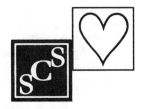

Epilogue

In the prologue to this book, we met Jeff, born in 1964, who had none of the advantages of a professional or lay public informed about fetal alcohol syndrome. It may seem that now we may know too much; that is, that there are expectations for all children known to be affected by prenatal alcohol and drugs. The exciting thing about intervention is that we never know how far we can take a particular child. The following letter written in response to published research about children and adults with fetal alcohol syndrome, points out the dangers thinking that we know all there is to know. It is worth sharing with the professional community to guard against such thinking.

> As the parent of a child diagnosed at birth as FAS, who is now in a pre-school speech and language class in our school district, I have become increasingly alarmed at the fatalism being spread regarding the learning "capacity" of my child from school district employees.
>
> Last spring, a physical therapist told me during a parent-teacher conference that "FAS children reach a learning plateau at the age of eight or nine." When school district officials were questioned about where they were getting this information they cited . . . [the current literature].
>
> However, according to a report issued by Lisa Pieper with the Alaska Council on the Prevention of Alcohol and Drug Abuse, in a March 1989 publication widely distributed in Interior Alaska, she quotes from . . . [a recent] study . . . as saying, "academic performance appears to peak at ages 12–15 (grades 6–8) and shows little improvement after this time."

Furthermore, her article states, "this pattern has led many experts to describe Fetal Alcohol Syndrome children as 'trainable but rarely educable.'"

The result of this reprint, as well as comments by local doctors and similar prevention publications found in school district offices has led to the perception among local educators that FAS children will not reach academic achievement above the third grade level.

As a result of this pervasive fatalism, an 8-year-old girl diagnosed as FAS was passed over in the selection of students eligible for limited tutorial services in favor of a child who "could benefit from additional assistance." The school instead opted to retain this girl in the third grade, although her only "failing" marks were in reading. The philosophy is apparently that achievement beyond this level is "highly unlikely."

Common sense tells us that children, like adults, will live up to the expectations set for them. Conversely, if those expectations are in truth limitations that tacitly prevent the child from reaching his full potential, a criminal disservice has been done to that individual.

When our son was born a "Fairbanks expert," on FAS warned us, as potential adoptive parents, that "an FAS baby will never be able to attend regular classrooms and will never be able to live independently if he reaches adulthood."

Upon our son's four month check-up, we were delighted as he demonstrated to the doctor that he could roll from back to stomach, which was pretty much on schedule for a child his age. Rather than rejoicing in this child's accomplishment, the doctor's response was to remind us that "you can't expect this child to function at age-appropriate skill levels." Hadn't he just exhibited an "age-appropriate skill"?

... The expectations, or rather limitations, now associated with an FAS diagnosis are rampant in our community. Everybody who has read even one article or has attended an hour-long workshop on FAS is suddenly an expert.

Our dentist made an FAS diagnosis of our son two minutes after meeting him. Anxious to share his wealth of information, he was quick to point out physical characteristics commonly associated with FAS, and proclaimed "he's hyperactive too, isn't he?"

A look of condescension and disbelief pouted his face when I responded that the child was not hyperactive. Neither his speech therapist of one year, his occupational therapist of two years, nor we as parents, have ever noted anything but an average amount of activity in our son. Yet again, a nurse was willing to attach that label to him shortly after an introduction because of the FAS diagnosis.

Just as educators and health technicians may be all too willing to assume that of course my child is hyperactive, I worry that these same people will also presume that his academic level will also bottom out at a given age, as some of . . . studies may or may not show.

. . . if your statistics are correct, we already have scores of FAS children in our school systems . . . Don't give [relatives and educators] a message of fatalism. Instead throw down the gauntlet of challenge to your audience to seek better methods of teaching these children . . . Don't allow the children of the 1990s to be limited to the accomplishments of those born two decades earlier.

If, together parents, community, and medical practitioners aren't able to exceed current expectations/limitations, then I suggest we're not trying — that we have in fact given up.[1]

---

[1] Reprinted with permission of Phyllis Tugman-Alexander.

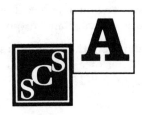

Appendix A
Infant-Parent
Interaction
Assessment

Bee, H. L., Barnard, K. E., Eyres, S. J., Gray, C. A., Hammond, M. A., Spietz, A. L., Snyder, C., and Clark, B. (1982). **Nursing Child Assessment Teaching and Feeding Scales.** In Prediction of IQ and language skill from perinatal status, child performance, family characteristics, and mother-infant interaction. *Child Development, 53,* 1134–1156.

Type of Measure: Behavioral checklist.

Purpose: Assessment of parent and child behaviors during teaching and feeding as a screening device and pre/post intervention.

Age Range: 1 to 36 months.

Source: From Sparks, S., Clark, M. J., Erickson, R. L., & Oas, D. B. (1990). *Infants at risk for communication disorders: Professionals' role in the home or center.* Tucson, AZ: Communication Skill Builders.

Content Areas: Parent's sensitivity to cues and response to distress, cognitive and socio-emotional growth fostering, and child's clarity of cues and responsiveness.

Administration Procedures: Check behaviors observed after 3 to 5 minutes of teaching; feeding observation time varies per dyad; rating time = 15 minutes per scale; 73/76-item binary checklist.

McCollum, J. A., and Stayton, V. D., (1985). **Social Interaction Assessment/Intervention.** In Studies and intervention guidelines based on the SIAI model. *Journal of the Division for Early Childhood, 9,* 125–135.

Type of Measure: Behavioral count.

Purpose: Evaluation of parent-handicapped child interaction pre/post intervention to increase parent's ability to make independent adjustments to child's behavior during play.

Age Range: Nonspecific.

Content Areas: Communicative social interaction; individualized target behaviors for parent and child, for example, imitation, vocalization, turn-taking.

Administration Procedures: Videotapes of 4-minutes of play in home; count target behaviors in 5–10 second intervals.

Owens, R. E. (1982). **Program for the Acquisition of Language with the Severely Impaired: The Diagnostic Interaction Survey and Caregiver Interview and Observation.** San Antonio, TX: The Psychological Corp.

Type of Measure: Informal caregiver interview and environmental observation.

Purpose: To identify the child's communication partners and the content, behaviors, and quality of child-caregiver communication.

Age Range: Nonspecific.

Robinson, E., and Eyberg, S. (1981). **Dyadic Parent-Child Interaction Coding System.** In the dyadic parent-child interaction coding system: Standardization and validation. *Journal of Consulting and Clinical Psychology, 49,* 245–250.

Type of Measure: Behavioral count.

Purpose: Assessment of degree to which parent's or child's behavior during play is deviant and evaluating effectiveness of treatment.

Age Range: Nonspecific.

Content Areas: Parent's directiveness, positive and negative physical contact; child's compliance.

Administration Procedures: Count behaviors during 5 minutes of play in clinic.

■ CAREGIVER ASSESSMENT

Bromwich, R. M., Khokha, E., Fust, L. S., Baxter, E., Burge, D., and Kass, E. W. (1978). **Parent Behavior Progression.** In Bromwich, R. (1981), *Working with parents and infants: An interactional approach.* Baltimore: University Park Press.

Type of Measure: Behavior checklist.

Purpose: Assessment of infant-related maternal behaviors to develop short-term goals aimed at changing maternal attitudes and behavior for the purpose of enhancing maternal-infant interaction.

Age Range: 2 forms: birth to 9 months, and 9 to 36 months.

Content Areas: Parent-infant relationship.

Administration Procedures: For use by practitioners familiar with family being assessed; establish rapport, observe spontaneous interaction, talk informally about activities with infant; after session with parent check behaviors on PBP if evidence from observation or parent report.

Field, R. M., Dempsey, J. R., Hallock, N. H., and Shuman, H. H. (1978). **The Mother's Assessment of the Behavior of Her Infant,** *Infant Behavior and Development, 1,* 156–157.

Type of Measure: Behavioral checklist for parents.

Purpose: To discern parental attitudes toward infant.

Age Range: Nonspecific.

Content Areas: Infant reactions to parental behaviors, crying, motor activities, physical characteristics.

Administration Procedures: Questions to parent about characteristics of infant.

Klein, M. D., and Briggs, M. H. (1987). **Observation of Communicative Interaction (OCI).** In Klein, M. D., and Briggs, M. H., Facilitating mother-infant communicative interactions in mothers of high-risk infants. *Journal of Communication Disorders, 10*(2), 95–106.

Type of Measure: Checklist.

Purpose: Evaluation of caregiver attributes.

Age Range: Nonspecific.

Content Areas: Provides tactile stimulation; pleasure; responses; positions; cues; modifications.

Administration Procedures: Observation of parent in interaction with infant.

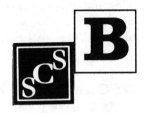

Appendix B
How To Get Help

■□ TELEPHONE HOTLINE NUMBERS

Cocaine Baby Help Line
1 (800) 638–BABY

To find out more about the harmful effects of cocaine on your unborn child and where to go for help.

Grandparents Warmline
(510) 568–7786
Mon. – Fri., 10:00 a.m. to 4:00 p.m.

For grandparents raising their grandchildren or greatgrandchildren to talk to other grandparents.

National Institute of Drug Abuse Hot Line
1 (800) HELP
9:00 a.m. to 3:00 p.m. EST

This help line is the only toll-free hot line available nationally to provide counseling and phone crisis intervention in addition to information services. Staff members are able to give names and numbers of treatment hospitals in an area that match a financial situation.

■□ INFORMATION FOR PARENTS AND PROFESSIONALS

National Perinatal Addiction Research and Education (NAPARE)
411 East Hubbard, Suite 200,
Chicago, IL 60611
(312) 329–2512

Memberships available. Members receive newsletter (*Perinatal Addiction Research and Education Update*) and discounts on conferences. Professional packets available to members and nonmembers.

National Council on Alcoholism and Drug Dependence
12 West 21st Street,
New York, NY 10010
1 (800) NCA–CALL
1 (800) 621–2155
9:00 a.m. to 5:00 p.m. EST

Has local affiliates in each state. They are usually listed in the telephone book as "(State Name) Council on Alcohol and Drug Dependence" or "National Council on Alcoholism Drug Dependence/(State Name)." Provides information packets, fact sheets, prevention brochures, and referral service. Some information on treatment and support groups. NCADD Fact Sheets: *Alcohol-Related Birth Defects*, available.

National Clearinghouse for Drug and Alcohol Abuse Information
P.O. Box 2345,
Rockville, MD 20852
(301) 468–2600
8:30 a.m. to 5:00 p.m. EST

Distributes publications by the National Institute on Drug Abuse (NIDA). Can do liteature searches on alcoholism and other drug issues. Can also provide referrals to other agencies and state clearinghouses on these topics.

Clearinghouse for Drug Exposed Children
Division of Behavioral and Developmental Pediatrics
University of California, San Francisco
400 Parnassus Avenue, Room A203
San Francisco, CA 94143-0314
(415) 476-9691

Resource and referral information for drug-exposed children and their
families. Newsletter.

March of Dimes
Local chapter or
March of Dimes Birth Defects Foundation
1275 Mamaroneck Avenue,
White Plains, NY 10605

Materials for parents and professionals.

Iceberg

Newsletter for parents and professionals to share information about FAS
and FAE. Iceberg, P.O. Box 4292, Seattle, WA 98104.

The Facts: "Alcohol-Related Birth Defects" and "Alcohol and Drugs"

Asha, The Journal of the American Speech-Language-Hearing Association, Supplement No. 6, to September 1991, *Asha, 33*(9), 34–35.

Cocaine/Crack: The Big Lie. DHHS (ADM) 87–1427, Revised 1987.

Superintendent of Documents, U.S. Government Printing Office, Washington, DC 20402. May be reproduced without permission.

■ VIDEOCASSETES

"What's Wrong With My Child?"
(March 30, 1990 episode of 20/20.)

Transcript available from Journal Graphics, 267 Broadway, New York,
NY 10007. (212) 732–8552. $4.00.
26 minute VHS available from Coronet MTI Film and Video, 108 Wilmot
Road, Deerfield, IL 60015. 1 (800) 621–2131. $295.

"Fetal Alcohol Syndrome"
(September 9, 1990. Episode No. 9013. Family Practice Update.)

Lifetime Medical Television, Box 5913 GPO New York, NY 10087.
(718) 482-4155. VHS. $54.13.

■□ AUDIOTAPE

"Fetal Alcohol Children in the Classroom"

Northwest Regional Educational Laboratory, P.O. Box 414, Portland, OR
97207. (503) 257–1515. $8.00 plus $3.00 handling, prepaid.

■□ BOOKS

Dorris, M. (1989). *The Broken Cord.* New York: Harper & Row, Inc.

A family's ongoing struggle with fetal alcohol syndrome. The story of an
adopted Indian boy with FAS written by his father. For parents and professionals. Hardback and paperback.

Villarreal, S. F., McKinney, L. E., & Quackenbush, M. (1992). *Handle with
Care: Helping Children Prenatally Exposed to Drugs and Alcohol*

Suggestions for parents, teachers, and other care providers of children to
age 10. Santa Cruz, CA: ETR Associates.

■□ CURRICULUM GUIDES

Children

Rice, K.S. et al. (1987). *Fetal Alcohol Syndrome Awareness Curriculum*

Available from: Ronald Reagan Resource Center for the Prevention of
Birth Defects, Meyer Children's Rehabilitation Institute, University of
Nebraska Medical Center, 444 South 44th Street, Omaha, NE 68131.
(402) 559–5700. 80 pp. $10.00.

A Manual on Adolescents and Adults with Fetal Alcohol Syndrome with Special Reference to American Indians

Available free from the Indian Health Service. Contact: Dr. George Brenneman, Maternal Child Health Coordinator, Indian Health Service, Parklawn Building, Room 6A-38, 5600 Fishers Lane, Rockville, MD 20857. (301) 443–1948.

Strategies for Teaching Young Children Prenatally Exposed to Drugs

Available from: School District of Hillsborough County, Linda B. Delapenha, M.S., 411 East Henderson Avenue, Tampa, FL 33602. (813) 272–4577.

Today's Challenge, Teaching Strategies for Working with Young Children Prenatally Exposed to Drugs/Alcohol

Available from: Valerie Wallace, Children Prenatally Exposed to Drugs, Los Angeles Unified School District, 450 North Grand Avenue, Suite H-120, Los Angeles, CA 90012.

Professionals

Alcohol and the Fetus: A Teaching Package

Available from: Fetal Alcohol Education Program, 7 Kent Street, Brookline, MA 02146. (617) 739–1424.

Taking a Drinking History (9 minutes) and *Counseling and Referral* (8 minutes)

Two films for training health professionals available from: Documentaries for Learning, 58 Fenwood Road, Boston, MA 02115. (617) 566–6793.

◼ WARNING POSTERS

"Alcohol Warning Signs: How to Get Legislation Passed in Your City"

$4.95 from Center for Science in the Public Interest, 1501 16th Street, NW, Washington, DC 20036. (202) 332–9110.

The following people can be contacted for information about warning posters.:

Mary Louise Frawley, 6404 Wilshire Boulevard, Suite 900, Los Angeles, CA 90048. (800) 421–3230.

Rick Kritzer, Prevention Coordinator, Alcoholism & Drug Abuse Programs. Columbus Health Department, 181 Washington Boulevard, Columbus, OH 43215-4096. (614) 222–7306.

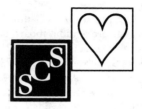

References

Abel, E. L., & Sokol, R. J. (1987). Incidence of fetal alcohol syndrome and economic impact of FAS-related anomalies. *Drug Alcohol Dependency, 19,* 51–70.

Ahmed, M. S., Spong, C. Y., Geringer, J. L., Mou, S. M., & Maulik, D. (1989). Prospective study on cocaine use prior to delivery. *Journal of the American Medical Association, 262*(13), 1880.

Ainsworth, M., Blehar, M., Waters, E., & Wall, S. (1978). *Patterns of attachment: A psychological study of the strange situation.* Hillsdale, NJ: Lawrence Erlbaum.

Allred, K. (1992). Fathers of young children with disabilities. *DEC* (Division for Early Childhood) *Communicator,* Council for Exceptional Children, *18*(3), 6–7.

Als, H., Duffy, F. H., & McAnulty, G. (in press). Neurobehavioral competence in healthy preterm and fullterm infants: Newborn period to 9 months. *Developmental Psychology.*

Als, H., Lester, B. M., Tronick, E., & Brazelton, T. B. (1982). Toward a research instrument for the assessment of preterm infants' behavior (APIB). In H. E. Fitzgerald, B. M. Lester, & M. W. Yogman (Eds.), *Theory and research in behavioral pediatrics* (Vol. 1, pp. 35–132). New York: Plenum Press.

American Psychiatric Association. (1987). *Diagnostic and statistical manual of mental disorders* (3rd ed., rev.). Washington, DC: American Psychiatric Association.

Anday, E. K., Cohen, M. E., Kelley, N. E., & Leitner, D. S. (1989). Effect of in utero cocaine exposure on startle and its modification. *Developmental Pharmacology and Therapeutics, 12*(3), 137–145.

Andrews, J. R., & Andrews, M. A. (1990). *Family based treatment in communicative disorders: A systematic approach.* Sandwich, IL: Janell.

Antoniadis, A., & Daulton, D. (1992). Meeting the needs of children in Pennsylvania who are exposed to alcohol and other drugs. *Infant-Toddler Intervention, 2*(1), 53–62.

American Medical Association. (1991). Drug abuse in the United States: Strategies for prevention. [Board of trustees report.] *Journal of the American Medical Association, 165*(16), 2102–2107.

Bagnato, S., & Neisworth, J. (1991). *Assessment for early intervention: Best practices for professionals.* New York: Guildford.

Bailey, D. B., & Simeonsson, R. J. (1988). Family needs survey. In D. B. Bailey & R. J. Simeonsson (Eds.), *Family assessment in early intervention.* Columbus, OH: Merrill.

Bailey, K. D. (1978). *Methods of social research.* New York: Free Press.

Bandura, A. (1977). *Social learning theory.* Englewood Cliffs, NJ: Prentice-Hall.

Bayley, N. (1969). *Bayley Scales of Infant Development.* New York: Psychological Corp.

Beardsley, B., Gillespie, T., & Williams, M. J. (1985, April). *Prevention of fetal alcohol syndrome/fetal alcohol effects: A comprehensive approach.* Paper presented at National Council on Alcoholism Conference, Washington, DC.

Beck, J. (1984, January 19). Will drinking harm your unborn baby? *Detroit Free Press,* p. 9A.

Becker, M., Warr-Leeper, G. A., & Leeper, H. A. (1990). Fetal alcohol syndrome: A description of oral motor, articulatory, short-term memory, grammatical, and semantic abilities. *Journal of Communication Disorders, 23,* 97–124.

Bennett, B. (1992, March). *Family issues: Women and the disease of addiction.* Paper presented at New Perspective on Substance-Exposed Infants Conference, Stanford University, Palo Alto, CA.

Black, M. (1991). Early intervention services for infants and toddlers: A focus on families. *Journal of Clinical Child Psychology, 20,* 51–57.

Blackman, J. (1984). Low birth weight. In J. Blackman (Ed.), *Medical aspects of developmental disabilities in children birth to three* (1st ed., rev.). Rockville, MD: Aspen.

Bloom, M. (1981). *Primary prevention: The possible science.* Englewood Cliffs, NJ: Prentice-Hall.

Blume, S. B. (1986). Women and alcohol: A review. *Journal of the American Medical Association, 256*(11), 1467–1470.

Botvin, G. J. (1983). Prevention of adolescent substance abuse through the development of personal and social competence: Preventing adolescent drug abuse. In T. J. Glynn, C. G. Leukefeld, & J. P. Ludford (Eds.), *NIDA Research Monograph 47* (pp. 115–140). Washington, DC: U.S. Department of Health and Human Services.

Brazelton, T. B. (1984). *Neonatal behavior assessment scale* (2nd ed.). Philadelphia: J. B. Lippincott.

Bryant, E. E., Kovar, M. G., & Miller, H. (1975). *A study of the effect of remuneration upon response in the health and nutrition examination survey.* In U.S. Department of Health, Education, and Welfare Publication No. (HRA) 76-1341, Series 2, Number 67, 1–18.

Burgess, D. M. (1990, May). *Fetal alcohol syndrome and fetal alcohol effect.* Presentation at National Council on Alcoholism of Michigan Workshop, Lansing.

Burgess, D. M., & Streissguth, A. P. (1990). Educating students with fetal alcohol syndrome or fetal alcohol effects. *Pennsylvania Reporter, 22*(1), 1–3.

Burgess, D. M., & Streissguth, A. P. (1992). Fetal alcohol syndrome and fetal alcohol effects: Principles for educators. *Phi Delta Kappan, 74,* 24–30.

Burns, K., Melamed, J., Burns, W., Chasnoff, I., & Hatcher, R. (1985). Chemical dependency and depression in pregnancy. *Journal of Clinical Psychology, 41,* 851–854.

Burns, W. J., & Burns, K. A. (1988). Parenting dysfunction in chemically dependent women. In I. J. Chasnoff (Ed.), *Drugs, alcohol, pregnancy and parenting* (pp. 159–171). Boston: Kluwer Academic Publishers.

Chasnoff, I. J. (1988). Introduction: The interfaces of perinatal addiction. In I. J. Chasnoff (Ed.), *Drugs, alcohol, pregnancy and parenting* (pp. 1–6). Boston: Kluwer Academic Publishers.

Chasnoff, I. J. (1991, June). President's message. *Perinatal Addiction Research and Education Update,* p. 1. (Available from National Association for Perinatal Addiction Research and Education, 411 Hubbard, Ste 200, Chicago, IL 60611.)

Chasnoff, I. J. (1991a). Methodologic issues in studying cocaine use in pregnancy: A problem of definitions. In M. M. Kilbey & A. Asghar (Eds.), *Methodological issues in controlled studies on effects of prenatal exposure to drugs* (DHHS Publication No. ADM 91-1837). Rockville, MD: U.S. Department of Health and Human Services.

Chasnoff, I. J. (1991b). Cocaine and pregnancy: Clinical and methodologic issues. *Clinics in Perinatology, 18*(1), 113–123.

Chasnoff, I. J. (1992a, March). *Cocaine in pregnancy.* Paper presented at New Perspective on Substance-Exposed Infants Conference, Stanford University, Palo Alto, CA.

Chasnoff, I. J. (1992b, May). *Drugs, alcohol, pregnancy and the child.* Paper presented at Drug Use in Pregnancy: Impact on Families and the Growing Child. National Association for Perinatal Addiction Research and Education (NAPARE) Conference, San Francisco.

Chasnoff, I. J., Burns, K. A., & Burns, W. J. (1987). Cocaine use in pregnancy: Perinatal morbidity and mortality. *Neurotoxicology and Teratology, 9,* 291–293.

Chasnoff, I. J., Burns, W. J., Schnoll, S. H., & Burns, K. A. (1985). Cocaine use in pregnancy. *The New England Journal of Medicine, 313*(11), 666–669.

Chasnoff, I. J., Griffith, D., Freier, C., & Murray, J. (1992). Cocaine/polydrug use in pregnancy: Two year follow-up. *Pediatrics, 89*(2), 284–289.

Chasnoff, I. J., Griffith, D. R., MacGregor, S., Dirkes, K., & Burns, K. A. (1989). Temporal patterns of cocaine use in pregnancy: Perinatal outcome. *Journal of the American Medical Association, 261*(12), 1741–1744.

Chasnoff, I. J., Landress, H. J., & Barrett, M. E. (1990). The prevalence of illicit-drug or alcohol use during pregnancy and discrepancies in mandatory report in Pinellas County, Florida. *New England Journal of Medicine, 322,* 1202–1206.

Chasnoff, I. J., Lewis, D. E., Griffith, D. R., & Wiley, S. (1989). Cocaine and pregnancy: Clinical and toxicological implications for the neonate. *Clinical Chemistry, 35*(7), 1276–1278.

Chavez, G. F., Cordero, J. F., & Becerra, J. E. (1989). Leading major congenital malformation among minority groups in the United States, 1981–1986. *Journal of the American Medical Association, 261,* 205–209.

Chavkin, W. (1991). Mandatory treatment for drug use during pregnancy. *Journal of the American Medical Association, 266*(11), 1556–1562.

Cherukuri, R., Minkoff, H., Feldman, J., Parekh, A., & Glass, L. (1988). A cohort study of alkaloidal cocaine ("crack") in pregnancy. *Obstetrics and Gynecology, 72*(2), 147–151.

Chouteau, M., Namerow, P. B., & Leppert, P. (1988). The effect of cocaine abuse on birth weight and gestational age. *Obstetrics and Gynecology, 72*(3), 351–354.

Church, M. W., & Gerkin, M. A. (1988). Hearing disorders in children with fetal alcohol syndrome: Findings from case reports. *Pediatrics, 82,* 147–154.

Clark, M. J., & Sparks, S. N. (1988). Evaluation of the at-risk infant. In D. Yoder & R. Kent (Eds.), *Decision making in speech-language pathology* (pp. 178–179). Toronto: B. C. Decker.

Clarren, S. K., & Smith, D. W. (1978). The fetal alcohol syndrome. *New England Journal of Medicine, 298,* 1063–1067.

Cohen, J. (1977). *Statistical power analysis for the behavioral sciences.* New York: Academic Press.

Cook, T. D., & Campbell, D. T. (1979). *Quasi-experimentation: Design and analysis issues for field settings.* Boston: Houghton Mifflin.

Coplan, J. (1984). *The early language milestone scale* (ELM). Tulsa, OK: Modern Education Corp.

Cregler, L., & Mark, H. (1986). Medical complications of cocaine abuse. *New England Journal of Medicine, 315,* 1495–1500.

Crites, L. S., Fischer, K. L., McNeish-Stengel, M., & Siegel, C. J. (1992). Working with families of drug-exposed children: Three model programs. *Infant-Toddler Intervention, 2*(1), 13–23.

Daghestani, A. N. (1988). Psychosocial characteristics of pregnant women addicts in treatment. In I. J. Chasnoff (Ed.), *Drugs, alcohol, pregnancy and parenting* (pp. 7–16). Boston: Kluwer Academic Publishers.

Dixon, S. D., Coen, R. W., & Crutchfield, S. (1987). Visual dysfunction in cocaine-exposed infants. *Pediatric Research, 21,* 359.

Donahue-Kilburg, G. (1992). *Family-centered early intervention for communication disorders: Prevention and treatment.* Rockville, MD: Aspen Press.

Dorris, M. (1989). *The broken cord.* New York: Harper & Row.

Finnegan, L. P. (1979). *Drug dependency in pregnancy: Clinical management of mother and child* (DHEW Publication No. ADM 79-678. Rockville, MD: Department of Health, Education and Welfare.

Finnegan, L. P. (1985). Neonatal abstinence. In N. M. Nelson (Ed.), *Current therapy in neonatal-perinatal medicine, 1985–1986* (pp. 262–270). St. Louis, MO: C. V. Mosby.

Fishbein, M., & Ajzen, I. (1975). *Belief, attitude, intention and behavior: An introduction to theory and research.* Reading, MA: Addison-Wesley.

Fisher, S. E. (1988). Selective fetal malnutrition: The fetal alcohol syndrome. *Journal of the American College of Nutrition, 7*(2), 417–421.

Forman, S. G., & Linney, J. A. (1988). School-based prevention of adolescent substance abuse: Programs, implementation and future directions. *School Psychology Review, 17*(4), 550–558.

Fulroth, R., Phillips, B., & Durand, J. J. (1989). Perinatal outcome of infants exposed to cocaine and/or heroin in utero. *American Journal of Diseases of Children, 143*(8), 905–910.

Furst, C. J., Beckman, L. J., Nakamura, C. Y., & Weiss, M. (1981). *Utilization of alcoholism treatment services.* Los Angeles: University of California at Los Angeles Alcohol Research Center.

GASP. (1992, March). *Bridging the gap.* Paper presented at New Perspective on Substance-Exposed Infants Conference, Stanford University, Palo Alto, CA.

George, W. H., & Marlatt, G. A. (1983). Alcoholism: The evolution of a behavioral perspective. In M. Galanter (Ed.), *Recent developments in alcoholism* (Vol. 1, pp. 105–138). New York: Plenum.

Giacoia, G. P. (1990). Cocaine in the cradle: A hidden epidemic. *Southern Medical Journal, 83*(8), 947–951.

Giunta, C. T., & Streissguth, A. P. (1988, September). Patients with fetal alcohol syndrome and their caretakers. *The Journal of Contemporary Social Work,* pp. 453–459.

Gold, S., & Sherry, L. (1984). Hyperactivity, learning disabilities and alcohol. *Journal of Learning Disabilities, 17*(1), 3–6.

Gomby, D. S., & Larson, C. S. (1992). Evaluation of school-linked services. *The Future of Children, 2*(1), 68–84.

Gomby, D. S., & Shiono, P. H. (1991). Estimating the number of substance-exposed infants. *The Future of Children, 1*(1), 17–25.

Goodstadt, M. S. (1978). Alcohol and drug education. *Health Education Monographs, 6,* 263–279.

Gordis, E. (1992, July 3). Fetal alcohol syndrome — A commentary by NIAAA director Enoch Gordis, M.D. *Alcohol Alert Supplement* (No. 12, PH 297). National Institute on Alcohol Abuse and Alcoholism.

Griffith, D. R. (1988). The effects of perinatal cocaine exposure on infant neurobehavior and early maternal-infant interactions. In I. J. Chasnoff (Ed.), *Drugs, alcohol, pregnancy and parenting* (pp. 105–113). Boston: Kluwer Academic Publishers.

Hadeed, A. J., & Siegel, S. R. (1989). Maternal cocaine use during pregnancy: Effect on the newborn infant. *Pediatrics, 84*(2), 205–210.

Hankin, J., & Firestone, I. (1992). Warning labels not dissuading some pregnant women on alcohol. *American Medical News, 35*(15), 24.

Hedrick, D. L., Prather, E. M., & Tobin, A. R. (1984). *Sequenced Inventory of Communication Development* (SICD). Seattle: University of Washington Press.

Henderson, G. I., & Schenker, S. (1977). Effects of ethanol and/or caffeine on fetal development and placental amino acid uptake in rats. *Developmental Pharmacology and Therapy, 7*(3), 177–187.

Hill, S. Y., & Smith, T. R. (1991). Evidence for genetic mediation of alcoholism in women. *Journal of Substance Abuse, 3,* 159–174.

Horgan, J. (1992). D_2 or not D_2: A barroom brawl over an "alcoholism gene." *Scientific American, 266*(4), 29–32.

Howard, J. (1989). Cocaine and its effects on the newborn. *Devopmental Medicine and Child Neurology, 31*(2), 255–257.

Howard, J., Beckwith, L., Rodning, C., & Kropenske, V. (1989). The development of young children of substance-abusing parents: Insights from seven years of intervention and research. *Zero to Three, 9*(5), 8–12.

Hume, R. F., O'Donnell, K. J., Stanger, C. L., Killam, A. P., & Gingras, J. L. (1989). In utero cocaine exposure: Observations of fetal behavioral state may predict neonatal outcome. *American Journal of Obstetrics and Gynecology, 161*(3), 685–690.

Institute of Medicine. (1990). Treating drug problems. In D. R. Gerstein & H. H. Harwood (Eds.), *A study of the evolution, effectiveness, and financing of public and private drug treatment systems* (Vol. 1, pp. 154–155). Washington, DC: National Academy Press.

Jaffe, J. H. (1990). Drug addiction and drug abuse. In L. S. Goodman & A. Gilman (Eds.), *The pharmacological basis of therapeutics* (8th ed., pp. 522–573). New York: Macmillan.

Jellinek, E. M. (1960). *The disease concept of alcoholism.* New Haven, CT: Hill-house Press.

Jones, C. L., & Lopez, R. (1990). Direct and indirect effects on infants of maternal drug abuse. In *Public Health Service report on the content of prenatal care* (Vol. 2). Washington, DC: Department of Health and Human Services/National Institutes of Health.

Jones, K. L., Smith, D. W., Streissguth, A. P., & Myrianthopoulos, N. C. (1974). Outcome in offspring of chronic alcoholic women. *Lancet, 1,* 1076–1078.

Kelly, J. G. (1979). 'Tain't what you do, it's the way that you do it. *American Journal of Community Psychology, 7*(3), 244–259.

Kenkel, W. (1966). *The family in perspective* (2nd ed.). New York: Appleton-Century-Crofts.

Klein, M. D., & Briggs, M. H. (1987). Facilitating mother-infant communicative interaction in mothers of high-risk infants. *Journal of Communication Disorders, 10*(2), 95–106.

Klein, M. D., & Briggs, M. H., & Huffman, P. A. (1988). *Facilitating caregiver-infant communication.* Los Angeles: California State University at Los Angeles, Division of Special Education.

Kronstadt, D. (1991). Complex developmental issues of prenatal drug exposure. *The Future of Children, 1*(1), 36–49.

Kumpfer, K. (1985). *Final report on the NIDA strengthening families program.* Salt Lake City: Social Research Institute, University of Utah.

Kumpfer, K. (1991). Treatment programs for drug-abusing women. *The Future of Children, 1*(1), 50–60.

Kumpfer, K., & Holman, A. (1985). *Women and substance abuse: A review.* Salt Lake City, UT: State Division of Alcoholism and Drugs.

Lester, B. (1984). Data analysis and prediction. In Brazelton, T. B. (Ed.), *Neonatal behavior assessment scale* (2nd ed.). Philadelphia: J. B. Lippincott.

Lester, B., Corwin, M. J., Sepkoski, C., Seifer, R., Peucker, M., McLaughlin, S., & Golub, H. L. (1991). Neurobehavioral syndromes in cocaine-exposed newborn infants. *Child Development, 62,* 694–705.

Lewis, K. D., Bennett, B., & Schmeder, N. H. (1989). The care of infants menaced by cocaine abuse. *Maternal Child Nursing, 14*(5). 324–329.

Little, B. B., Snell, L. M., Klein, V. R., & Gilstrap, L. C. (1989). Cocaine abuse during pregnancy: Maternal and fetal implications. *Journal of Obstetrics and Gynecology, 73*(2), 157–160.

Little, B. B., Snell, L. M., & Rosenfeld, C. R. (1990). Failure to recognize fetal alcohol syndrome in newborn infants. *American Journal of Diseases of Children, 144,* 1142–1146.

Little, R. E. (1977). Moderate alcohol use during pregnancy and decreased infant birthweight. *American Journal of Public Health, 67*(12), 1154–1156.

Little, R. E., & Streissguth, A. P. (1982). Alcohol: Pregnancy and the fetal alcohol syndrome. In *Alcohol Use and Its Medical Consequences: A Comprehensive Teaching Program for Biomedical Education* (Unit 5). [Slide teaching unit.] Project Cork of Dartmouth Medical School. (Available from Milner-Fenwick, Inc., 2125 Greenspring Drive, Timonium, MD 21093.)

Little, R. E., & Wendt, J. K. (1991). The effects of maternal drinking in the reproductive period: An epidemiologic review. *Journal of Substance Abuse, 3,* 187–204.

Little, R. E., Young, A., Streissguth, A. P., & Uhl, C. M. (1984). Preventing fetal alcohol effects: Effectiveness of a demonstration project. In *Mechanisms of alcohol damage in utero* (CIBA Foundation Monograph No.105). London: Pitman.

MacGregor, S. N., Keith, L. G., Chasnoff, I. J., Rosner, M. A., Chisum, G. M., Shaw, P. D., & Minogue, J. P. (1987). Cocaine use during pregnancy: Adverse perinatal outcome. *American Journal of Obstetrics & Gynecology, 144,* 23–27.

Marshall, A. B. (1991, September). State-by-state legislative review. *Perinatal Addiction Research and Education Update,* p. 1–3. (Available from National Association for Perinatal Addiction Research and Education, 411 Hubbard, Ste 200, Chicago, IL 60611.)

Mayes, L. C., Granger, R. H., Bornstein, M. H., & Zuckerman, B. (1992). The problem of prenatal cocaine exposure: A rush to judgment. *Journal of the American Medical Association, 267*(3), 406–408.

McBride, W. G. (1977). Thalidomide embryopathy. *Teratology, 16,* 79–82.

McCormick, M. C., Brooks-Gunn, J., Workman-Daniels, K., Turner, J., & Peckham, G. J. (1992). The health and developmental status of very low-birthweight children at school age. *Journal of the American Medical Association, 267*(16), 2204–2208.

McKim, W. A. (1991). *Drugs and behavior: An introduction to behavioral pharmacology* (2nd ed.). Englewood Cliffs, NJ: Prentice-Hall.

McNagy, S. E., & Parker, R. M. (1992). High prevalence of recent cocaine use and the unreliability of patient self-report in an inner-city walk-in clinic. *Journal of the American Medical Association, 267*(8), 1106–1108.

Miller, G. (1989). Addicted infants and their mothers. *Zero to Three, 9*(5), 20–23.

Minor, M. J., & Van Dort, B. (1982). Prevention research on the teratogenic effects of alcohol. *Preventive Medicine, 11,* 346–359.

Mirriam, S. (1988). *Case study research in education: A qualitative approach.* San Francisco: Jossey-Bass.

Morse, B., Weiner, L., & Garrido, P. (1989). Focusing prevention of fetal alcohol syndrome on women at risk. *Annals of the New York Academy of Sciences, 562,* 342–343.

Multiclinic. (1991). *Multiclinic 88.* [Videotape.] Kalamazoo: Western Michigan University Media Services.

Murray, A. (1992). Early intervention program evaluation: Numbers or narratives? *Infants and Young Children, 4*(4), 77–88.

National Council on Alcoholism and Drug Dependence (NCADD). (1990). *Women, alcohol, other drugs and pregnancy.* [Policy statement.] (Available from NCADD. 12 West 21st St., New York, NY 10010.)

National Institute on Alcohol Abuse and Alcoholism. (1981). In J. R. DeLuca (Ed.), *Fourth special report to the U.S. congress on alcohol and health* (DHHS Publication No. ADM 82-1080, p. 36). Rockville, MD: U.S. Department of Health and Human Services.

National Institute on Drug Abuse. (1991). *National Household Survey on Drug Abuse: Main Findings, 1990* (DHHS Publication No. ADM 91-1788). Rockville, MD: U.S. Department of Health and Human Services.

Norris, J., & Hoffman, P. (in press). *Whole language intervention for school-age children.* San Diego: Singular Publishing Group.

O'Brien, C. P. (1976). Experimental analysis of conditioning factors in human narcotic addiction. *Pharmacological Reviews, 27,* 533–543.

Ostrea, E. M., Parks, P., & Brady, M. (1989). The detection of heroin, cocaine, and cannabinoid metabolites in meconium of infants of drug dependent mothers. *Annals of the New York Academy of Sciences, 562,* 373–374.

Phibbs, C. S., Bateman, D. A., & Schwartz, M. (1991). The neonatal costs of maternal cocaine use. *Journal of the American Medical Association, 226*(11), 1521–1526.

Phillips, D. K., Henderson, G. I., & Schenker, S. (1989). Pathogenesis of fetal alcohol syndrome. *Alcohol Health and Research World, 13*(3), 219–227.

Pickens, R. W., & Svikis, D. S. (1991). Genetic influences in human substance abuse. *Journal of Addictive Diseases, 10*(1/2), 205–213.

Randall, T. (1991). Intensive prenatal care may deliver healthy babies to pregnant drug abusers. *Journal of the American Medical Association, 265*(21), 2773–2774.

Randall, T. (1992). Infants, children test positive for cocaine after exposure to second-hand crack smoke. *Journal of the American Medical Association, 267*(8), 1044–1045.

Rawson, R. A., Obert, J. L., McCann, M. J., Castro, F. G., & Ling, W. (1991). Cocaine abuse treatment: A review of current strategies. *Journal of Substance Abuse, 3,* 457–491.

Riley, E. P., & Vorhees, C. V. (1986). *Handbook of behavioral teratology.* New York: Plenum.

Rinkel, P. (1992, June). Myths and stereotypes about long-term effects of prenatal alcohol and other drug exposure (PADE). *Perinatal Addiction Research and Education Update,* p. 1–3. (Available from National Association for Perinatal Addiction Research and Education, 411 Hubbard, Ste 200, Chicago, IL 60611.)

Rist, M. C. (1990). The shadow children. *The American School Board Journal, 177*(1), 19–24.

Rivers, K. O., & Hedrick, D. L. (1992). Language and behavorial concerns for drug-exposed infants and toddlers. *Infant-Toddler Intervention, 2*(1), 63–73.

Roberts, R., Wasik, B., Casto, G., & Ramey, C. (1991). Family support in the home: Programs, policy, and social change. *American Psychology, 46,* 131–137.

Rodning, C., Beckwith, L., & Howard, J. (1990, March). *Characteristics of attachment organization and play organization in prenatally drug-exposed toddlers.* Paper presented at the Workshop on Children and Parental Illicit Drug Use: Research, Clinical and Policy Issues. Washington, DC: National Research Council, Institute of Medicine.

Ronan, L. (1985). State strategies for prevention of alcohol-related birth defects. *Alcohol Health and Research World, 10*(1), 60–65.

Rosenstock, I. M. (1974). Historical origins of the Health Belief Model. *Health Education Monographs, 2,* 328–335.

Rosenstock, I. M. (1990). The health belief model: Explaining health behavior through expectancies. In K. Glanz, F. M. Lewis, & B. K. Rimer (Eds.), *Health behavior and health education: Theory research and practice* (pp. 39–62). San Francisco: Jossey-Bass.

Rosett, H. L. (1979). Clinical pharmacology and the fetal alcohol syndrome. In E. Majchrowitz & E. P. Noble (Eds.), *Biochemistry and pharmacology of ethanol* (Vol. 2, pp. 485–510). New York: Plenum.

Rosett, H. L., Weiner, L., & Edelin, K. C. (1983). Treatment experience with pregnant problem drinkers. *Journal of the American Medical Association, 249*(15), 2029–2033.

Roth, P. (1991, November). *Women, alcohol and addiction.* Paper presented at A Seminar on Current Prevention, Treatment and Policy Issues, National Council on Alcoholism of Michigan, Lansing.

Rundall, T. G., & Bruvold, W. H. (1988). A meta-analysis of school-based smoking and alcohol use prevention programs. *Health Education Quarterly, 15*(3), 317–334.

Samaroff, A., & Chandler, M. J. (1975). Reproductive risk and the continuum of caretaking casualty. In F. D. Horowitz, M. Hetherinton, S. Scarr-Salapatek, & G. Siegel (Eds.), *Review of child development research,* (Vol. 4, pp. 187–244). Chicago: University of Chicago Press.

Schafer, W. (1989). President's column. *The Infant Crier, 49,* 2. (Available from Michigan Association for Infant Mental Health, Department of Psychology, Michigan State University, East Lansing, MI 48824.)

Schafer, W. (1990). President's column. *The Infant Crier, 50,* 1–2. (Available from Michigan Association for Infant Mental Health.)

Schafer, W. (1991). President's column. *The Infant Crier, 55,* 1–2. (Available from Michigan Association for Infant Mental Health.)

Schultz, F. R. (1984). Respiratory distress syndrome. In J. Blackman, (Ed.), *Medical aspects of developmental disabilities in children birth to three* (1st ed., rev., pp. 207–209). Rockville, MD: Aspen.

Serdula, M., Williamson, D. F., Kendrick, J. S., Anda, R. F., & Byers, T. (1991). Trends in alcohol consumption by pregnant women: 1985 through 1988. *Journal of the American Medical Association, 265*(7), 876–879.

Shaywitiz, S., Cohen, D., & Shaywitz, B. (1980). Behavior and learning difficulties in children of normal intelligence born to alcoholic mothers. *Journal of Pediatrics, 96,* 978–982.

Smith, C. A. (1947). Effects of maternal undernutrition upon the newborn infant in Holland. *Journal of Pediatrics, 30,* 229–243.

Snowden, L. R., Munoz, R. F., & Kelly, J. G. (1979). *Social and psychological research in community settings.* San Francisco: Jossey-Bass.

Sokol, R. J., Miller, S. I., & Reed, G. (1980). Alcohol abuse during pregnancy: An epidemiologic review. *Alcoholism: Clinical and Experimental Research, 4*(2), 134–145.

Sparks, S. (1989). Assessment and intervention with at-risk infants and toddlers. In G. Ensher & S. Sparks (Eds.), Early intervention: Infants, toddlers and families. *Topics in Language Disorders, 10*(1), 43–56.

Sparks, S. (1990). *A synthesis review of behaviors displayed by neonates with antenatal cocaine exposure.* Unpublished paper.

Sparks, S., Clark, M. J., Erickson, R. L. & Oas, D. B. (1990). *Infants at risk for communication disorders: Professional's role with the newborn.* Tucson AZ: Communication Skill Builders.

Sparrow, S. S., Balla, D. A., & Cicchetti, D. V. (1984). *Vineland Adaptive Behavior Scales.* Circle Pines, MN: American Guidance Service.

Stewart, J., de Wit, H., & Eidelboom, R. (1984). Role of unconditioned and conditioned drug effects in the self-administration of opiates and stimulants. *Psychological Review, 91*(2), 251–268.

Strategies for teaching young children prenatally exposed to drugs. (1990). Drug exposed children's committee. Tampa, FL: Hillsborough County Public Schools.

Streissguth, A. P. (1990, May). *Fetal alcohol syndrome and fetal alcohol effect.* Paper presented at National Council on Alcoholism of Michigan Workshop, Lansing.

Streissguth, A. P., Aase, J. M., Clarren, S. K., Randels, S. P., LaDue, R. A., & Smith, D. F. (1991). Fetal alcohol syndrome in adolescents and adults. *Journal of the American Medical Association, 265,* 1961–1967.

Streissguth, A. P., Barr, H. M., Sampson, P. D., Parrish-Johnson, J. C., Kirchner, G. L., & Martin, D. C. (1986). Attention, distraction and reaction time at age 7 years and prenatal alcohol exposure. *Neurobehavioral Toxicology and Teratology, 8,* 717–725.

Streissguth, A. P., Clarren, S. K., & Jones, K. L. (1985). Natural history of the fetal alcohol syndrome: A ten-year follow-up of eleven patients. *Lancet, 2,* 85–92.

Streissguth, A. P., & Giunta, C. T. (1988). Mental health and health needs of infants and preschool children with fetal alcohol syndrome. *International Journal of Family Psychiatry, 9*(1), 29–47.

Streissguth, A. P., Herman, C. P., & Smith, D. W. (1979). Intelligence, behavior and dysmorphogenesis in the fetal alcohol syndrome: A report on 20 patients. *The Journal of Pediatrics, 92*(3), 363–367.

Streissguth, A. P., & LaDue, R. (1985). Psychological and behavioral effects in children prenatally exposed to alcohol. *Alcohol and Health Research World, 10,* 6–12.

Streissguth, A. P., & LaDue, R. (1987). Fetal alcohol: Teratogenic causes of developmental disabilities. In S. Schroeder (Ed.), *Toxic substances and mental retardation* (pp. 1–32). Washington, DC: American Association on Mental Deficiency.

Streissguth, A. P., LaDue, R., & Randels, S. P. (1988). *A manual on adolescents and adults with fetal alcohol syndrome with special reference to American Indians.* Seattle: University of Washington.

Streissguth, A. P., Landesman-Dwyer, S., Martin, J. C., & Smith, D. W. (1980). Teratogenic effects of alcohol in humans and laboratory animals. *Science, 209,* 353–361.

Streissguth, A. P., & Randels, S. (1988). Long term effects of fetal alcohol syndrome. In G. C. Robinson & R. W. Armstrong (Eds.), *Alcohol and child/family health* (pp. 135–151). Vancouver: University of British Columbia.

Streissguth, A. P., Sampson, P. D., & Barr, H. M. (1989). Neurobehavioral dose-response effects of prenatal alcohol exposure in humans from infancy to adulthood. *Annals of the New York Academy of Sciences, 562,* 145–158.

Streissguth, A. P., Sampson, P. D., & Barr, H. M., Darby, B. L., & Martin, D. C. (1989). IQ at age 4 in relation to maternal alcohol use and smoking during pregnancy. *Developmental Psychology, 215*(1), 3–11.

Summers, J., Dell'Oliver, C., & Turnbull, A. (1990). Examining the individualized family service plan process: What are family and practitioner preferences? *Topics in Early Childhood Special Education, 10,* 78–99.

Tarr, J. E., & Macklin, M. (1987). Cocaine. *Pediatric Clinics of North America, 34,* 319–331.

The Future of Children. (1992). Appendix B: Evaluation in a sample of current school-linked service efforts, *2*(1), 142–143.

Thiel, S., Nelson, K., Alrick, J., & Brodsky, M. (1977). *Social skills and sex education guide.* Salem: State of Oregon, Department of Developmental Disabilities.

Today's challenge: Teaching strategies for working with young children prenatally exposed to drugs/alcohol. (1989). [Pamphlet.] Los Angeles: Los Angeles Unified School District.

Trout, M., & Foley, G. (1989). Working with families of handicapped infants and toddlers. *Topics in Language Disorders, 10*(1), 56–67.

University of Nebraska Medical Center News. (1988). Counseling program hopes to prevent fetal alcohol syndrome. *9*(1), 11.

U.S. General Accounting Office Report to the Chairman, Committee on Finance, U.S. Senate. (1990). *Drug exposed infants: A generation at risk* (GAO/HRD Publication No. 90-138).

VanBremen, J. (1991, June). Defining at-risk children under public law 99-457, a NAPARE survey. *Perinatal Addiction Research and Education Update,* pp. 1–3. (Available from National Association for Perinatal Addiction Research and Education, 411 Hubbard, Ste. 200, Chicago, IL 60611.)

VanBremen, J. (1992, May). *Drug use in pregnancy: Impact on families and the growing child.* Paper presented at the National Association for Perinatal Addiction Research and Education (NAPARE) Conference, San Francisco.

VandenBurg, K. A. (1985). Revising the traditional model: An individualized approach to developmental intervention in the intensive care nursery. *Neonatal Network, 4,* 32–56.

Vorhees, C. V., & Butcher, R. E. (1982). Behavioral teratogenicity. In K. Snell (Ed.), *Developmental toxicology* (pp. 247–298). New York: John Wiley.

Vuchinich, R. E., & Tucker, J. A. (1988). Contributions from the behavioral theory of choice to an analysis of alcohol abuse. *Journal of Abnormal Psychology, 97,* 181–195.

Weiner, L., Rosett, H. L., & Mason, E. A. (1985). Training professionals to identify and treat pregnant women who drink heavily. *Alcohol Health & Research World, 10*(1), 32–35.

Werner, E., & Smith, R. (1982). *Vulnerable but invincible.* New York: McGraw-Hill.

Weston, D. R., Ivins, B., Zuckerman, B., Jones, C., & Lopez, R. (1989). Drug exposed babies: Research and clinical issues. *Zero to Three, 9*(5), 1–7.

Wilson, J. G. (1977). A new area of concern in teratology. *Teratology, 16,* 227–228.

Yancosek, K. B. (1982). *Better beginnings for babies.* [Program manual for Pennsylvania Project for Prevention of Fetal Alcohol and Drug Effects.] (Available from Washington-Greene Prevention Corporation, Washington, PA.)

Zuckerman, B. (1991). Drug-exposed infants: Understanding the medical risk. *The Future of Children, 1*(1), 26–35.

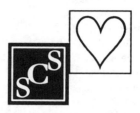

Index